Preface to First Edition.

This work, as its title suggests, is a companion to the author's "Essentials of Homœopathic Materia Medica."

The latter was a quiz compend of the Principles of Homœopathy, Homœopathic Pharmacy and Homœopathic Materia Medica, while the present work is a quiz compend of the application of Homœopathic remedies to diseased states in like manner systematized, condensed and simplified especially for the use of Students of Medicine.

The "Essentials of Homœopathic Therapeutics" should, therefore, go hand in hand with its predecessor, since it will enable the student concisely to perfect his knowledge, not alone in the science of Homœopathic Materia Medica, but, what is still more important, in the practical application of such knowledge to diseased conditions.

One of the grand cardinal features of Homœopathy and one little understood by the Allopathic school is the fact that any drug in the entire Homœopathic Materia Medica may be a remedy in any diseased state. It is therefore evident that the preparation of this work entailed no little difficulty, and that many remedies may be missed where they would seem naturally to find a place. Especially have remedies indicated in diseases by their well-known general characteristic symptoms been omitted. For instance; *Arsenicum* is sometimes a remedy in Pneu-

Preface to Second Edition.

The call for a second edition of this little work within so short a time after the appearance of the first, leads the author to congratulate himself that it actually found the place in homœopathic literature for which it was designed, namely, a companion to the "*Essentials of Homœopathic Materia Medica.*" While its title is *Therapeutics*, it should be looked on by the student simply as *Materia Medica* in another form. If this be done there is little danger of the student falling into the practice of the ancient school of associating remedies with diseases, or diagnosis with treatment.

The universal favorable criticism bestowed upon the first edition encourages the author to hope that the present one in its thoroughly revised shape may receive the same approval.

Not only has the work been thoroughly revised and numerous errors, which appeared in the first edition corrected, but also the size has been necessarily increased by the addition of many characteristic indications.

W. A. DEWEY, M. D.

Ann Arbor, Mich., June 15, 1897.

monia, but the symptoms calling for use, such as extreme prostration, restlessness, pale face, periodicity, irregular pulse, red tongue, etc., belong to many diseased conditions, and would indicate *Arsenicum* wherever found; therefore *Arsenicum* has been omitted as a remedy in Pneumonia.

Comparisons of remedies in diseased conditions have sometimes made it necessary to depart from a strict alphabetical arrangement of the remedies; for quizzing purposes this is of little import, and for those who may use the work for reference the difficulty will be easily overcome by consulting the index, which it has been the intention to make complete.

W. A. DEWEY, M. D.

New York, October 25, 1894

CONTENTS.

Abortion,	1
Abscess	1
Acne,	3
After Pains,	4
Agalactia,	5
Alcoholism,	6
Amenorrhœa,	7
Anæmia,	9
Angina Pectoris,	11
Aphonia,	136
Aphthæ,	180
Apoplexy,	12
Appendicitis,	12
Asthma,	13
Backache,	15
Boils,	18
Bones, Diseases of,	19
Brain, Diseases of,	20
Bright's Disease,	147
Bronchitis,	22
Cancer,	238
Carbuncle,	26
Chlorosis,	9
Cholera Asiatica,	27
Cholera Infantum,	29
Chorea,	32
Climateric Disorders,	33
Colds and Catarrhs,	34
Colic,	42
Constipation,	44
Convulsions,	49
Coryza,	34
Coughs,	51
Croup,	57
Cystitis,	244
Debility,	59
Delirium,	60
Delirium Tremens,	6
Dentition,	61
Diabetes,	62
Diarrhœa,	62
Diphtheria,	73
Dropsical Affections,	75
Dysentery,	77
Dysmenorrhœa,	78
Dyspepsia,	95
Ears, Diseases of,	80
Eczema,	213
Eneuresis,	243
Epilepsy,	82
Epistaxis,	116
Erysipelas,	85
Eye, Diseases of,	86
Fever, Simple,	92
Fever, Typhoid,	237
Fissure of Anus,	94
Gangrene,	95
Gastric Derangements,	95
Glandular Troubles,	110
Gleet,	111
Gonorrhœa,	112
Gout,	114

CONTENTS.

Hay Fever,	115
Hemorrhages,	116
Hemorrhoids,	119
Headaches,	121
Heart, Affections of,	130
Herpes,	213
Hoarseness,	136
Hydrocephalus,	138
Hysteria,	139
Influenza,	141
Injuries,	142
Intermittent Fever,	144
Insomnia,	221
Insanity,	165
Iritis,	86
Kidney, Diseases of,	147
Labor,	148
Laryngitis,	150
Leucorrhœa,	151
Liver, Diseases of,	153
Loco-Motor Ataxia,	158
Lumbago,	15
Mammary Gland, Affections of,	160
Marasmus,	161
Measles,	162
Meningitis,	164
Mental Conditions and Derangements,	165
Menstrual Disorders,	251
Miscarriage,	179
Mouth, Diseases of,	180
Mumps,	181
Neuralgia,	182
Neuræsthenia,	184
Ophthalmia,	86
Orchitis,	185
Otitis,	80
varian Diseases,	187
Ozæna,	34
Paralysis,	188
Parotitis,	181
Peritonitis,	189
Phthisis,	190
Pleurisy,	193
Pleurodynia,	193
Pneumonia,	194
Pregnancy, Diseases of,	199
Puerperal State,	201
Rheumatism,	202
Scarlet Fever,	208
Sciatica,	210
Scrofula,	211
Seasickness,	212
Skin, Diseases of,	212
Sleeplessness,	221
Sore Throat,	223
Spermatorrhœa,	227
Spinal Irritation,	226
Spleen, Diseases of,	231
Sunstroke,	231
Synovitis,	232
Syphilis,	232
Teeth, Affections of,	234
Tetanus,	235
Tonsillitis,	236
Tumors,	237
Typhoid Fever,	237
Ulceration,	242
Urinary Disorders,	243
Vertigo,	247
Vomiting,	248
Whooping Cough,	249
Women, Diseases of,	251
Worms,	261
Yellow Fever,	262

HOMŒOPATHIC THERAPEUTICS.

ABORTION.

(See Miscarriage.)

ABSCESS.

What remedy is most often indicated in the beginning of Abscess? Give the symptoms.

Belladonna. The parts are bright red, the swelling appears suddenly and is rapid, the pus developing with lightning-like rapidity. There is a throbbing sensation which is intense and sudden and the pains are apt to cease as suddenly as they appeared. Acute abscesses.

Wherein do Hepar Sulphur, Calcium sulphide and Calcarea sulphurica differ in chemical composition?

Hepar is a combination of flowers of sulphur and lime from the middle layer of the oyster shell. It is an impure Sulphide of Calcium.

Calcium sulphide is the chemically pure article.

Calcarea sulphurica is the Sulphate of Calcium or Gypsum.

Give indications for these three remedies in Abscess.

Hepar when there are chills indicating beginning of suppuration, with throbbing and sharp sticking pains; given low in threatening suppuration it favors it, but given high it will often abort it.

Calcium sulphide is a make-shift for Hepar, it has not been proved.

Calcarea sulphurica has not been thoroughly proved, but clinically it has been found useful in cases of abscess where the suppuration is prolonged. The presence of pus with a *vent* is an indication. It comes in after *Silicea*.

When is Silicea indicated in suppuration?

In conditions where the suppuration continues and the wound refuses to heal; the process is an indolent and a sluggish one. The discharge is apt to be thin and watery.

How does Silicea differ from Calcarea sulphurica in the suppurative process?

Silicea promotes suppuration and brings the suppurative process to maturity. *Calcarea sulphurica* checks suppuration and promotes healthy granulation. It lacks also the fetor of *Silicea*.

When should Mercurius be given in Abscess?

It is indicated after *Belladonna*, when pus has formed and needs to be evacuated. It favors the rapid formation of pus. Glandular abscesses especially call for *Mercurius*. There is intense shining redness, with throbbing and stinging pains.

What are the relations of Mercurius and Silicea?

They do not follow each other well, hence must be carefully distinguished.

Give indications for Lachesis in Abscess.

In low conditions of abscess when the pus is thin, dark, and offensive in character. The inflamed parts are purplish in color. Abscesses from poisonous matter introduced into the system.

When should Sulphur be given?

In chronic cases when the discharge is profuse, with emaciation and hectic fever. Abscesses in scrofulous persons where there is a marked psoric taint.

What are some other remedies especially useful in Scrofulous abscesses?

Calcarea carb., and if about the glands of the neck *Calcarea iod.*

Besides Lachesis, what remedies may be indicated in low conditions of Abscess by general symptoms?

Arsenic, *Rhus tox.* and *Carbo veg.*

What external applications are useful and non-compatible with Homœopathic treatment?

The application of heat, as poultices or hot water, relaxes and soothes the parts and favors the formation and discharge of pus.

ACNE.

(See also Skin, Diseases of.)

What remedy is most often called for in Acne, and what are its indications?

Sulphur; the skin is harsh and rough; the acne is principally on the face and is associated with comedos. Great aggravation from water.

When is Sanguinaria indicated in Acne?

Especially in women who have scanty menses and irregular circulation of blood.

Give indications for Ledum.

Red, pimply eruption on the face; small pimples at the root of the nose; acne in brandy drinkers.

What are the remedies for Acne due to sexual excesses, masturbation, etc.?

Antim. crud., *Aurum*, *Phosphoric acid* and *Kali brom.*

What are some other remedies that may be found indicated in Acne?

Natr. mur., *Antim. tart.* and *Hepar.*

What local applications may be used?

Hot water is the least injurious. Thorough washing with Castile soap and hot water is the best treatment. Under no condition should medicated applications be used.

AFTER PAINS.

What are the indications for Cimicifuga in After Pains?

When they are very intense; worse about the region of the groin and the patient is sensitive and cannot tolerate them. Rheumatic subjects.

When should Caulophyllum be given?

When the labor has been prolonged and the pains are

spasmodic across the lower part of abdomen. Also an excellent remedy for false labor pains.

Give another remedy which has been verified in After Pains.

Xanthoxylum.

Give a few other remedies for After Pains.

Chamomilla, Pulsatilla, Arnica, Crocus, Belladonna and *Gelsemium.*

Why should After Pains not be checked at once?

After pains are caused by nature's efforts to expel clots of blood or portions of membrane from the uterus, which are necessary to perfect involution.

AGALACTIA.

Give indications for Pulsatilla in this affection.

The breasts are swollen, painful, and the flow of milk is absent or scanty. The patient is depressed and tearful.

Give a remedy often used for non-appearance of milk, without apparent cause.

Urtica urens.

When is Chamomilla indicated in suppression of milk?

When the suppression results from a fit of anger.

What other remedies may be thought of?

Ricinus communis or castor oil, *Agnus cast.*, *Belladonna* and *Calcarea*.

ALCOHOLISM.

Give indications for Nux vomica in Alcoholism.

Morning vomiting, trembling of hands, nervous affections, bad taste in mouth, headache. Constant uneasiness and troublesome visions.

When is Hyoscyamus indicated?

When there is a constant loquacious delirium, small, quick and compressible pulse, cold and clammy skin; delirium tremens.

When is Opium indicated in Mania-a-Potu, or Delirium Tremens?

In old "sinners" whose constitution is a wreck and who have had repeated attacks of the disease. There is a constant expression of fright or terror; they have visions of animals springing up everywhere, see ghosts, and sleep is disturbed; breathing is stertorous; it is especially applicable to those cases which simulate apoplexy.

Mention some other drugs having the symptoms of frightful images, animals, etc., and how are they distinguished?

Lachesis. Visions of snakes and hideous objects; sensation in throat as if choking; waking suddenly out of sleep.

Stramonium has visions of animals approaching him from every corner; tries to escape; bright red face.

Arsenicum. Visions of ghosts and fanciful figures with trembling and weakness; diseased from over-use of alcohol; must have their accustomed drink.

What remedy. clinically, has been found to exert a beneficial effect on the maniacal attacks of drunkards?

Ranunculus bulbosus.

Give indications for Sulphuric Acid in Alcoholism.

Inebriates who are on their "last legs;" they are pale, shriveled and cold, and their stomachs will not tolerate the slightest amount of food; cannot drink water unless it contains whiskey. Their manner is quick and hasty in everything. It comes in long after *Nux vomica*. Great craving for brandy.

What remedies have been used successfully in combatting the craving for spirituous liquors?

Sulphur, *Nux vom.* and *Arsenicum*.

AMENORRHŒA.

What drugs have suppression of menses from violent emotions such as fright, etc.?

Aconite, *Lycopodium*, *Opium*, and *Veratrum*.

Give indications for Calcarea carb. in menstrual suppression.

First menses are delayed, and there is apt to be congestion about head and chest; there is palpitation of the heart, dyspnœa worse when ascending, and headache. In scrofulous subjects and those with cold, damp feet, who perspire easily about the head.

How does Belladonna come in here?

With *Belladonna* there is a rush of blood to head, throbbing in temples, subjective feeling of coldness and

8 ESSENTIALS OF

feeling of weight and fulness in pelvis; much bearing down.

Give indications for Pulsatilla, which is a useful remedy in a majority of cases.

Amenorrhœa caused by getting feet wet is the characteristic, with general *Pulsatilla* symptoms and conditions.

What other drug has Amenorrhœa from getting the feet wet?

Dulcamara. This drug is characterized further by an eruption on the skin at each menstrual period.

What are the indications for Ferrum in delayed menses?

Delayed first menses with debility, languor, palpitation, sickly complexion and puffiness about ankles.

Mention two drugs useful for vicarious menstruation and give some indications therefor.

Bryonia. Epistaxis in place of menstrual discharge; dry cough; oppression of chest and heaviness of head; symptoms all worse from motion.

Phosphorus. Spitting and vomiting of blood at menstrual periods; especially useful in tall, slender, phthisical subjects.

Give indications for Apis in Amenorrhœa.

Congestion to head and bearing down in uterine region. Hysterical, nervous and awkward with flushing of face, or a puffy, waxy condition; pains in right ovary.

When might Cimicifuga be useful in Amenorrhœa?

When the menses are irregular, tardy or suppressed and accompanied by reflex nervous disturbances.

Mention a few other remedies that may be useful in Amenorrhœa.

Graphites, *Sepia*, *Sulphur*, and *Natrum mur*.

What auxiliary measures may be used in this affection?

Hot sitz baths and hot water injections; these are especially indicated where the suppression is caused by exposure to cold or getting wet, and there is bearing down in pelvis.

ANÆMIA.

When is Ferrum met., the great anæmic remedy, indicated in this trouble?

When the patient has the appearance of full bloodedness or plethora, which is followed by a paleness and earthiness of the face and puffiness of the extremities.

When is Cinchona indicated in Anæmia?

When caused by loss of fluids, as from long-continued diarrhœa or hemorrhage, a condition when the quantity and quality of the blood is changed.

In what similar condition is Calcarea phosphorica useful?

In chlorosis or the "green sickness." The face is white, pale or sallow, or waxy and greenish, and the menses are apt to be too early.

Give symptoms of Pulsatilla, another remedy in anæmic and chlorotic conditions.

After abuse of iron and quinine the system is relaxed and the patient feels worn out, is constantly chilly and she suffers from uterine and menstrual derangements. It will often be the first remedy to use if the case comes from allopathic hands.

What is a clinical use of Ferrum aceticum?

In stubborn anæmia and debility. In children who grow tall rapidly and are so active that they become easily exhausted; they keep thin, weak and pale.

Give indications for Ferrum phosphoricum in Anæmia.

It is useful to improve the quality of the red blood corpuscles and follows *Calcarea phosphorica* well, but should be indicated by general symptoms.

When is Natrum mur. indicated?

Anæmia from loss of fluids. Especially in women who suffer from menstrual disorders; blood is impoverished.

When is Alumina a remedy in anæmic and chlorotic conditions?

When they occur at puberty, and there is an abnormal craving for indigestible substances, as slate pencils, chalk, etc.

Give indications for Graphites.

Mucous membranes pale. Throbbing on lying down at night; tendency to a rush of blood to head.

ANGINA PECTORIS.

What are the symptoms of Cimicifuga in this affection?

The pains radiate all over the chest and there is a sensation as if the left arm were bound to the side.

Give indications for Arsenicum.

Patient must sit up; holds his breath, it being painful to breathe. Pains radiate from heart all over chest; cold sweat, weak, scarcely perceptible pulse and burning about heart.

When is Glonoine the remedy?

Where there is fluttering and violent beating of the heart, as if the chest would burst open, labored breathing and radiating pains.

When should Amyl nitrite be given?

Where there is constriction about the heart and oppressed breathing and where the slightest thing causes flushing; it is an important remedy for the immediate relief of the paroxysm.

Give indications for Spigelia.

Anguishing, substernal pain, radiating to neck and arms; irregular pulse; tendency to syncope, palpitation, and severe stabbing stitches in heart.

Mention some remedies for the condition known as "Tobacco heart."

Nux vomica, *Tabacum*, *Kalmia* and *Gelsemium*.

APHONIA.

(See Hoarseness.)

APHTHÆ.

(See Mouth, Diseases of.)

APOPLEXY.

What are the indications for Opium in Apoplexy?

Rattling, stertorous breathing, and a very dark red face, and sometimes a tetanic rigidity of the body and paralysis; the darker red the face the more it is indicated.

When would Arnica be called for?

When there is aching soreness all over the body. Bed sores form readily. Paralysis, especially on left side, full and strong pulse and stertorous breathing.

When there are convulsions accompanying, what remedies should be thought of?

Belladonna, Hyoscyamus and *Lachesis*.

Give some indications for Belladonna.

The effusion is attended with symptoms of violent congestion; if given early may be of use. Pupils are dilated, face flushed, throbbing of carotids.

When should Gelsemium be used?

In threatened apoplexy with a general relaxed state of the system, weakness and trembling; muscles refuse to obey the will.

APPENDICITIS.

What are the indications for Belladonna in this affection?

Pain in ileo-cæcal region. Cannot bear slightest touch; worse by jar, motion of bed or turning of body. Patient lies on back. Fever and general symptoms, such as flushed face, etc., are present.

When is Rhus indicated?

There is a hard, painful swelling of the right side of abdomen, pain worse when sitting or stretching right leg. Cannot lie on left side.

Give indications for Bryonia.

Pain dull and throbbing or sharp and sticking, confined to a limited spot. Patient is constipated.

Give symptoms of Lachesis.

Pain and swelling in region of cæcum. Pain extends from right lumbar region, through inguinal region and fore part of thigh. Patient weak.

Give two drugs that have been found of great service clinically in this affection.

Ferrum phos., and *Kali mur*.

ASTHMA.

What is an indication for the use of Ammoniac gummi?

Humid asthma, with tenacious expectoration and a sensation as if something would be torn loose.

Give indications for Arsenicum.

Attacks of suffocation, especially at night or when lying down; great anguish and restlessness. Cannot lie down for fear of suffocation. Especially useful if the disease be chronic and the dyspnœa habitual.

In what respiratory affection is Natrum sulphuricum useful?

In asthma. In asthma which is worse upon change to damp weather. Moist asthma, with a great deal of rattling on the chest. The shortness of breath is especially worse in damp weather. Looseness of bowels at each attack, worse from alcohol. Sycotic taint.

What are the indications for Stramonium in Asthma?

In nervous asthma, where the voice suddenly gives out and takes on a higher pitch. Great sense of suffocation with tight feeling across chest; face becomes blue.

What are the symptoms of Ipecac in this affection?

Spasmodic asthma, with weight and anxiety about the chest; sudden wheezing dyspnœa, threatening suffocation; aggravated by motion; the cough causes gagging and vomiting.

What are the symptoms of Lobelia inflata in Asthma?

There is a weak sensation in epigastrium extending up into chest; nausea; profuse salivation; great oppression of chest, relieved by moving about; sensation of lump in stomach; attacks preceded by a prickly sensation through the whole system.

Give indications for Kali bichromicum.

Worse at three or four o'clock in the morning; relieved by raising stringy mucus; relief also from sitting up and bending forward.

Mention three other drugs useful in asthmatic conditions that have peculiar symptoms.

Apis. He does not see how he can get another breath.

Bromine. Patient feels as if he could not get air enough into his lungs, consequently breathes very deeply. This is owing to constriction of glottis.

Grindelia. On falling asleep ceases to breathe and wakes with a start. Humid asthma and acute catarrhal asthma are sometimes benefited by this remedy.

What drug is useful in Asthma which is reflex from accumulation of gas in the stomach?

Carbo veg.

When is Nux vomica the remedy in Asthma?

When brought on by gastric disturbance, fulness and oppression worse after hearty meal; must loosen clothing; relieved by belching.

What other drug may be used for Asthma of gastric origin?

Zingiber. With this drug there is no anxiety.

What is the unique indication for Pothos in Asthma?

Asthma brought on or made worse from inhalation of dust of any kind.

BACKACHE.

Give the Backache of Æsculus.

Backache during pregnancy where the pain is in the sacro-iliac synchondroses, and that part of the back gives out, compelling her to sit.

What is the Backache of Calcarea fluorica?

Backache simulating spinal irritation; pain in the lower

part of the back with a fulness or burning pain. Lumbago worse on beginning to move, and relieved by continued motion. Lumbago from strains.

What symptoms has Kali phosphoricum in the back?

There is rheumatic lameness of the back, which is worse after rest and on just commencing to move; they are especially worse on rising from a sitting position; there seems to be a paralytic tendency.

What drug has these same symptoms?

Rhus tox.

What drug has stiffness in the lumbar region with a sudden loss of power on attempting to move?

Sulphur.

What is the Backache of Oxalic acid?

Acute pain in the back extending down the thighs, relieved by change of posture: the back feels too weak to support the body; the pains are worse when thinking of them.

What symptoms has Phosphorus in the back that are characteristic?

Intense burning pains in the spine between the scapulæ; the dorsal spines are very sensitive.

Give the indications for Rhus in Lumbago.

Pain in back on attempting to rise; rheumatic pains in the back and stiff neck from sitting in a draft; the lumbago is a condition which may not be relieved by motion and still indicate *Rhus*.

What drugs have Backache worse while sitting?

Cobalt, Zincum, Sepia, and *Cannabis Ind.*

When is Ledum indicated in Backache?

There is a stiffness of the back as after sitting a long time.

What drugs have pains in the lumbar region compelling the patient to get up and walk about?

Staphisagria and *Kali carb.*

What drugs are useful for rheumatic pains in the back which are worse in the morning before rising?

Petroleum and *Ruta.*

What drugs have a stiff back which is worse when first beginning to move?

Anacardium and *Conium.*

What is a remedy for a sudden kink or catch in the back?

Secale.

What remedy has the symptom that the patient cannot turn over in bed without first sitting up on account of rheumatic pains in back?

Nux vomica.

What is the Backache of Nux?

In the lumbar region; worse at night when lying in bed; cannot turn over without sitting up; lumbago.

BOILS.

When is Arnica the remedy in Boils?

It produces crops of boils all over body, beginning with great soreness and going on to suppuration. Boils which have partially matured become sluggish.

In Boils when is Belladonna useful?

When they are very painful. Swellings where there is throbbing, redness and tendency to suppuration.

When is Calcarea sulph. indicated?

When there is great swelling and tumefaction and the boil is discharging.

When should Silicea be given?

In boils which occur in crops and do not heal readily, but continue to discharge a thin pus; areola indurated.

When is Hepar to be preferred in Boils?

Where there is much throbbing and sticking in them. In the early stages if given high it will sometimes abort them, if given low it will favor the ripening process.

Give indications for Lachesis.

The surface is very sensitive, bluish, and the central sore is apt to be surrounded by many small pimples.

Give three remedies most useful for a disposition to Boils.

Calc. carb., *Lyc.* and *Sulphur*.

BONES, DISEASES OF.

What are the Bone symptoms of Asafœtida?

Periosteal inflammations and ulcerations; the ulcers are sensitive and intolerant to dressings; the discharge is offensive.

Give the indications for Calcarea fluorica in Bone diseases.

Hard, rough, corrugated elevations on bones, bruises of bones; caries, leading to the formation of pelvic abscesses, affections of nasal bones, caries from syphilis or abuse of Mercury.

What action has Calcarea phosphorica on the Bones?

It has an action at the places where the bones form a suture or joint; it is also useful to favor the uniting of fractures, hastening the formation of callus.

What are the symptoms of Fluoric acid on the Bones and periosteum?

It produces caries of the long bones, with thin and excoriating discharges, relieved by cold applications. Dental fistulæ and bone felons, with offensive discharges.

When is Silicea indicated in Bone troubles?

In scrofulous children whose bones are curved, spinal curvature; Potts' disease; fistulous tracks running to diseased bone.

How does Phosphorus compare?

It is useful in Necrosis, especially of the lower jaw; also caries.

Mention some other drugs useful in Caries.

Platina mur. Caries of the Tarsus; *Angustura*, especially of the long bones; *Strontiana carb.*, of the femur; *Aurum*, cranial bones and bones of nose and palate after abuse of Mercury; pains aggravated by touch; burning pains, worse at night; excessively fetid discharges.

What remedy is useful for injuries of the bones?

Symphytum off.

What remedy is useful in Syphilitic affections of the long bones?

Stillingia.

BRAIN, DISEASES OF.

When is Aconite useful in Cerebral affections?

Idiopathic cerebral inflammation, cerebral congestion from anger or exposure to sun.

Give indications for Belladonna.

Congestion to the head, face red, or it may be pale, eyes injected, throbbing headache; is drowsy or wakeful. Jerking of limbs. Sharp, shooting pains, forcing patient to cry out; they come suddenly and disappear suddenly; dilated pupils. Grinding of the teeth; often convulsions.

How is Belladonna distinguished from Glonoine in Cerebral affections?

They are quite similar. *Glonoine* is worse from bending head backwards, *Belladonna* better; *Glonoine* better by motion, *Belladonna* worse; *Glonoine* relief from uncovering head, *Belladonna* relief from covering head.

HOMŒOPATHIC THERAPEUTICS. 21

What drugs have the symptom of a swashing feeling in the Brain when moving about?

Cinchona, Carbo an., Belladonna, Spigelia, Rhus tox., and *Sulphuric acid.*

What are the Cerebral symptoms of Hyoscyamus?

Delirium, prostration and stupor, open mouth, dropped jaw. Cerebral inflammation with pulsating waves through the head; relieved by shaking head or sitting with head bent forward. (*Belladonna* opposite.)

What symptoms referring to the brain call for Kali bromatum?

Brain fag, benumbed feeling in the brain, sensation as if about to lose senses—caused by overwork.

Give indications for Phosphorus in softening of the brain.

Dull pain in head; wearied, tired feeling and difficulty in walking.

When is Nux vomica indicated in Brain affections?

Cerebral softening due to sedentary habits and intemperance. Vertigo in the morning. Vacillating gait, headache when exciting mind. Brain fag, with gastric symptoms.

Mention two other drugs useful in Brain Fag.

Picric acid and *Phosphoric acid.*

Give cerebral symptoms of Stramonium.

Violent delirium, restlessness, screaming out as if terrified, grinding of teeth, etc.

When is Zincum useful in Brain affections?

When the brain becomes affected in the course of nervous diseases, scarlatina, or summer complaints; paralysis from softening of brain following suppressed foot sweat.

What are the cerebral symptoms of Veratrum viride?

Cerebral hyperæmia with febrile condition; headache, throbbings of carotids, flushed face; full, hard, bounding pulse.

BRIGHT'S DISEASE.

(See Kidneys, Diseases of,)

BRONCHITIS.

When is Aconite the remedy in this disease?

At the commencement when due to checked perspiration. It mitigates the dry cough, lessens the fever and prevents extension of capillary congestion.

Give indications for Belladonna in Bronchitis.

There is tickling in the larynx and a dry, hacking cough, which is paroxysmal; dryness and tightness in the upper part of the chest, worse evenings and at night; the larynx is sore and hot.

In what affections of the chest is Natrum muriaticum useful?

In chronic bronchial catarrhs, winter coughs and asthma, where there is a profuse secretion of mucus.

When is Ammonium carb. indicated in Bronchitis?

Where there is copious accumulation of mucus in the lungs. The patient is weak, coughs continually, but raises little. There is congestive fulness and rawness of the chest with discharge of bluish, slate colored mucus, and rattling of large bubbles of mucus in the chest.

Give indications for Causticum in Bronchitis.

Deep hollow dry cough, with pain in the chest, especially under sternum. Rattling in chest when coughing, with soreness. Tightness of chest; must take a deep breath, often involuntary spurting of urine when coughing.

What remedies are useful for bronchial Catarrh with profuse expectoration?

Balsam peru, and *Pix liquida*.

What are the indications for Bryonia in Bronchitis?

Pressure over sternum, great dyspnœa, dry cough, seeming to start from stomach, worse after a meal; pains in sides.

What are the respiratory symptoms of Carbo vegetabilis?

Evening hoarseness, with rawness and scraping in the larynx and trachea; oppression of chest; bronchitis in old people when there is a loose rattling in the chest on coughing or breathing. Profuse yellow, fetid expectoration; bronchial hemorrhage.

What is the action of Ipecac in bronchial affections?

There is a dry spasmodic cough, ending in choking and gagging, and a tickling which extends from the larynx to the extremities of the bronchi; coarse rales all over the chest, with violent paroxysms of coughing and retching, face pale and great dyspnœa; incessant cough with every breath.

How do these symptoms compare with Antimonium tart.?

Fine rales, but very little cough, increased dyspnœa, weakness and drowsiness; the chest seems full of mucus, but they cannot cough it up.

What other remedy has a similar symptom to the latter, and is especially applicable to old people?

Baryta carb.

What are the indications for Chelidonium?

Capillary bronchitis following measles or whooping cough with hepatic symptoms, oppression of the chest, fan-like motion of the alæ nasi, and one hot and one cold foot. The cough is loose and rattling, and the expectoration is not easily raised.

What other drug has as characteristics a fan-like motion of the alæ nasi, a hot foot and a cold one?

Lycopodium.

Give symptoms of Kali bichromicum.

Bronchitis, especially if glands be involved. The expectoration is of thick, tenacious, viscid mucus; it can be drawn into strings to the feet; worse from eating; relieved when warm in bed; croupy cough, hoarseness, with pains in the epigastrium.

What are the symptoms of Kali carbonicum in Bronchitis?

Intense dyspnœa, cough worse at two or three in the

morning; there are stitching pains through the lower part of the right lung, accompanied by puffiness of the face; much mucus on chest; the expectoration is difficult and tenacious, or of small round lumps.

Give the respiratory symptoms of Kali sulphuricum.

There is a cough, with great *rattling of mucus* on the chest; the cough is worse in a warm room, and relieved in the cool, open air. The rattling may occur with or without much cough.

Give indications for Lycopodium in bronchial Catarrh.

Where the smaller tubes are affected, much mucus, rales, rattling breathing, cough and dyspnœa; expectoration yellowish and thick; right lung more affected.

Give in brief the indications for Phosphorus.

Cough worse on going from warm into cold air. Dry, tickling cough, caused by laryngeal or sub-sternal irritation; tearing pain under sternum, as if something were torn loose. Suffocative pressure across upper part of the chest. Expectoration is yellowish and blood streaked. It is largely the bronchial symptoms that indicate *Phosphorus* in pneumonia.

What are indications for Sanguinaria?

Burning in the chest; dry, hacking cough and feeling of dryness in the air passages. Oppression of breathing and a tenacious, difficult expectoration, which is apt to be rust colored; there are also sharp stitching pains through the right lung.

When is Sulphur indicated in bronchial affections?

Chronic bronchitis where there is a large accumulation.

of thick muco-pus. Patient has suffocative spells. Loud râles through the chest.

CANCER.

(See Tumors.)

CARBUNCLE.

Give indications for Arsenicum in Carbuncle.

Carbuncle, where there are lancinating and burning pains; worse after midnight; relieved by heat.

When would Anthracinum be found indicated in Anthrax or Carbuncle?

Where the symptoms are the same as under *Arsenicum*, only more intense; pains cutting and lancinating, and *Arsenicum* has failed to relieve.

Give the indications for Lachesis in Carbuncles.

When there is great sensitiveness of the surface, bluish appearance and perhaps the central sore surrounded by many small pimples; carbuncles which slough and are very offensive.

Give indications for Rhus in Carbuncle.

There is formation of pus, intense pain and dark red swelling, with the general prostration of the remedy.

What is the use of Tarentula Cubensis?

It produces a perfect picture of sloughing carbuncle with great prostration, and it relieves the atrocious pains accompanying it.

When should Carbo veg. be used?

When the affected parts are bluish; when the discharge is offensive, tends to become gangrenous. It lacks the restlessness of *Arsenic*, though burning pains are present.

CHLOROSIS.

(See Anæmia.)

CHOLERA ASIATICA.

What are the indications for Camphor in Cholera?

Body cold as ice; great prostration; voice squeaky or husky; upper lip retracted; indicated more at the beginning without any vomiting or diarrhœa. Tongue, nose and ears are cold; collapse, with scanty or absent discharges.

Give symptoms indicating Carbo vegetabilis in state of collapse.

Icy coldness of the body; cold breath; bluish countenance, and a desire for air; coldness of the legs to the knees is very characteristic; the collapse in *Carbo vegetabilis* is due to the drain on the system from the discharges.

What are the indications for Cuprum in Cholera?

Coldness and blueness of the surface of the body, cramps of the muscles, those of the calves and thighs are drawn up into knots; there is distress in the pit of the stomach and great dyspnœa.

What are the symptoms of Secale in Cholera?

Retching and vomiting of undigested food, body wasted and cold, cramps, tingling in limbs, face sunken, mouth distorted; profuse, painless discharge from the bowels, ejected with violence; cold, clammy sweat.

How does Secale differ from Arsenicum in Cholera?

Both have profuse, offensive, watery stools. *Arsenicum* lacks the tingling of *Secale*, and wants to be warmly wrapped up. *Secale* wants to be cool and lacks the anxious tossing about and restlessness of *Arsenicum*.

What other drug besides Camphor has sudden cessation of all discharges and collapse?

Hydrocyanic acid.

Give another remedy which produces a perfect picture of Cholera.

Jatropha.

Is Aconite ever useful in Cholera?

In cholera when collapse comes on very rapidly with little or no premonitory illness, unattended by copious evacuations.

What are the symptoms indicating Veratrum in Cholera

Profuse, watery, greenish like spinach, or bloody stools, with cramps and cutting pains in the abdomen and limbs, with great weakness and fainting; little vomiting, cold sweat on the forehead and rice-water stools, attended with prostration and collapse; aggravation at night; pale face, sunken eyes, and prostration.

How does this differ from Camphora?

Camphora has coldness without sweat; the tongue is cold; the discharges are scanty; the upper lip is retracted, showing the teeth; the voice is high pitched and the entire body is cold.

When should one give Cuprum?

When the cramps are very severe and extend to the chest; vomiting and purging, but lacking the cold sweat of *Veratrum*.

CHOLERA INFANTUM.

What is the characterizing indication for Aconite in this affection?

Stools looking like chopped spinach. Febrile conditions.

When is Argentum nitr. indicated?

Green, slimy stools with noisy flatus, worse at night, in thin, dried up children, who look like mummies.

Give indications for Arsenicum.

Stools undigested, worse after eating or drinking and after midnight, with rapid emaciation and weakness.

When is Belladonna suitable?

In yellowish-green stools, containing lumps looking like caseine. Erethism and tendency to cerebral trouble.

Give indications for Bismuth.

Watery, offensive and painless stool with much rumbling in bowels during stool. After stool child is exhausted. Much gagging, but child only vomits when stomach is full.

What is the Summer Complaint of the Calcarea child?

Craving for eggs; milk disagrees; it is vomited in cakes and curds; milk is sometimes passed in this condition also. Diarrhœa worse towards morning, of green, undigested, watery, sour stools.

How does Calcarea phos. compare?

Here there is craving for bacon and ham; there is great emaciation; the stools are green, slimy and accompanied with much flatus.

Give briefly the chief indications for Croton tig.

Yellow, watery stools; a little pain, then forcible expulsion and aggravation from eating or drinking.

Give indications for Ferrum phos.

Frequent, watery stools; child becomes rapidly reduced and falls into a stupor.

What drug has watery, olive green stools coming out with a gush?

Elaterium.

When is Ipecac indicated?

In the commencement; nausea and vomiting of everything eaten or drunk; stools green or yellow and liquid, and covered with mucus and blood.

What is the characteristic of Podophyllum in Cholera?

Absence of pain; stools are watery, profuse, come out with a gush; loathing of food; worse in morning.

How does Aethusa compare?

Aethusa stools are without odor, and vomiting does not prevent the child from nursing or feeding, which is opposite to *Podophyllum*.

Give in brief symptoms of Psorinum in Cholera Infantum.

Nervous and restless at night; awake frightened or cry out during sleep. Diarrhœa; profuse, watery stools, dark brown, even black; very offensive; almost putrid; worse at night.

When is Sulphur indicated?

Diarrhœa worse towards morning; ravenous hunger; greenish, watery, offensive stools; flabby abdomen.

Give briefly the indications for Veratrum.

Profuse, watery stools, preceded by abdominal pain and followed by great prostration.

Give indications for Chamomilla.

Child cross and fretful, wants to be carried; greenish-yellow stool; colic, child draws up its knees; moaning in sleep.

When should China be thought of?

Watery, undigested stool, which is profuse and painless; rapid emaciation; worse after eating.

Give symptoms calling for Mercurius.

Green, frothy or yellow stools, or bloody with straining and desire to sit after stool.

CHOREA.

What are the indications for Agaricus in Chorea?

Angular choreic movements; itching of the eyelids and of various parts of the body as if they had been frost bitten; diminished intellect, almost imbecility. Blepharospasmus, twitching of the eyelids and eyeballs.

What are the indications for Magnesia phosphorica in Chorea?

It is a useful remedy in chorea, with contortions of the limbs; also in cramps, such as writers' cramps, piano or violin players' cramps. Spasmodic twitching of eyelids or facial muscles.

In what affection is Mygale lasiodora used?

In chorea, where there are twitchings of the facial muscles, irregular convulsive movements of one side of the body; the words are jerked out; the movements cease during sleep, but return more violent in the morning.

What remedy is useful for choreic movements due to uterine troubles?

Cimicifuga.

Mention four other drugs useful in Chorea?

Tarentula, Ignatia, Zizia and *Stramonium.*

When is Zincum indicated in Chorea?

When it is caused by fright or suppressed eruptions, especially when there is great depression of spirits, and when the general health suffers greatly.

Give indications for Causticum.

Right side; words are jerked out on attempting to speak; legs and arms "on the go" during sleep.

CLIMACTERIC DISORDERS.

What climacteric symptoms does Lachesis correspond to?

The headache, and the fact that non-appearing discharges make the patient worse; flushes of heat during the day.

Give indications for Glonoine.

When the flushings of heat are confined to the head, and there is much throbbing.

Give the use of Sanguinaria during the climacteric.

Flushes of heat, flatulent distention of stomach, leucorrhœa fetid and corrosive, menses offensive, profuse; uterine polypi. Breasts sore, palpitation, acne, burning in hands and feet.

Give another drug indicated in flushes of heat during change of life.

Amyl nitrite.

What are the disorders calling for Cimicifuga?

Sinking at epigastrium, pain on top of head, great irritability of disposition and pain in left side.

COLDS AND CATARRHAL AFFECTIONS.

When is Aconite indicated in commencing colds?

When the attack comes on suddenly after exposure to dry cold winds, and there is chilliness followed by fever; no discharge, nose dry and stopped up; symptoms all better in the open air.

When does Camphora suit these colds in the head?

In the first stage, where the nose is stuffed up and the febrile symptoms of *Aconite* are wanting, though the patient feels chilly; there is depression and languor. An indicating symptom is that the inspired air feels cold.

When should we give Gelsemium?

There is a general malaise and a feeling as if a cold were coming on; the head is hot and full and there is chilliness and a disposition to hug the fire; colds from relaxing weather; there is a watery, bland discharge from the nose and sneezing.

When is Arsenic indicated in colds?

Where there is a thin, watery discharge from the nose, which excoriates the upper lip, and in spite of this fluent discharge the nose feels stopped up; the patient is chilly and hugs the fire; there is frontal headache, photophobia and sneezing, and the sneezing does not relieve the irritation in the slightest; it is worse going into the open air, though the burning is worse near the fire.

How does this differ from Mercurius?

The *Mercurius* discharge, though very excoriating, is not watery, but thicker; it is a thin, mucous discharge.

How does Arsenicum differ from Phosphorus in colds?

The cold of *Arsenicum* always settles in the nose, while that of *Phosphorus* settles in the chest.

How do we differentiate Allium cepa here?

Allium cepa has excoriating nasal discharge, but there is profuse lachrymation which is bland; there is prolonged sneezing; the discharge ceases on going into the open air, but returns again when coming into a warm room.

What are the characteristics of Sabadilla?

Influenza with violent spasmodic sneezing and lachrymation on going into the open air; burning, watery discharge from the nose; eyes swollen and watery; swelling of the throat and tonsils. Hay fever. Chilly, sensitive to cold air, wants to be wrapped up; sneezes when inhaling cold air; desires hot drinks.

What other drug has a thin, watery discharge from the nose, and how is it differentiated from the foregoing?

Euphrasia; it has excoriating lachrymation and bland nasal discharge, just the opposite of *Allium cepa*. The cough of *Euphrasia* has been described as "measly."

What are the indications for Arum triphyllum in colds?

There is a stopped up nose with a fluent, acrid discharge, which is most generally yellow, and there is much soreness of the nostrils.

Mention another drug which has stoppage of the nose with a discharge.

Lycopodium; here there is apt to be posterior dryness; discharge of yellowish green matter from nose anteriorly.

In the first stages of colds when should Ferrum phos. be given?

When the onset of a cold is less sudden than that calling for *Aconite* and where there is no anxiety or restlessness.

When is Nux vom. indicated in cold in the head?

In the first stage, when brought on by damp, cold weather, sitting on damp steps, etc., associated with sneezing and stuffed up feeling in the nose. The nose is dry, very little discharge; the eyes water; there is scraping in the throat, and there is dullness and oppression in the frontal region; the symptoms are worse in a warm room and better in the open air.

How does Mercurius compare?

It is similar in the rawness and soreness in the nose, and it is worse in damp weather.

Compare also Arsenicum.

The coryza is relieved by warmth and aggravated by cold, which is the opposite of *Nux*, and the discharge is very thin and burning.

What other drug has distress in the frontal region with excoriating coryza, lachrymation, etc.?

Kali hydriodicum; here all discharges are profuse and watery, and the throat is irritated. Patient is alternately hot and cold.

Give indications for Natrum mur. in colds.

Watery discharges, which are accompanied by vesicular eruptions about the lips, mouth and nose, dryness of the posterior nares and loss of smell and taste; sneezing worse in the evening while undressing and in morning on rising.

What is the difference between Sinapis nigra and Arsenicum?

Sinapis has the heat of *Arsenicum*, but there is dryness in the nose and no discharge.

What are the nasal symptoms of Chamomilla?

The nose is stopped up, yet runs a watery mucus; sneezing and inability to sleep; a dry, teasing cough keeping the child awake, or else a rattling cough, as if the bronchi were full of mucus.

Give catarrhal symptoms of Mercurius.

Profuse coryza extending to the frontal sinuses, with burning in eyes and nose; the discharge is a thin mucus, not thick nor yet watery, but excoriating; worse in damp weather; ulceration with acrid discharge.

What drugs have specially watery discharges?

Allium cepa, *Arsenic*, *Euphrasia*, *Arum triphyllum*, *Kali hyd.* and *Natrum mur*.

Mention some drugs with thick discharges from the nose.

Pulsatilla, *Cyclamen*, *Penthorum*, *Kali bich.*, and *Hydrastis*.

What are the symptoms calling for Pulsatilla in colds?

A ripe cold with a thick, yellow and bland discharge, no sneezing or excoriation, simply a thick, yellow mucopurulent discharge which is bland.

Supposing that we have these same symptoms and in addition a great deal of sneezing, what is the remedy?

Cyclamen.

ESSENTIALS OF

What would indicate Penthorum sedoides?

The same symptoms as *Pulsatilla*, but in addition a rawness in the throat and a feeling of wetness in the nose.

Give the symptoms indicating Hydrastis in Nasal catarrh.

Watery, excoriating coryza, with burning and rawness in the nose and a sensation as if a hair were in the nose, the discharge being more profuse out of doors; later a thick, yellow, tenacious discharge and a constant dropping from the posterior nares into the throat.

How does this condition differ from that found under Kali bich.?

With *Kali bich.* there is a tendency to deep ulceration, and the mucus is even more tenacious and stringy than under *Hydrastis*.

Is there any ulceration with Hydrastis?

There is, but it is a more superficial ulcerative process than that under *Kali bich*.

Is Spigelia ever indicated in Catarrh?

It is useful where the mucus passes off only through the posterior nares.

What are the indications for Kali bich. in Catarrh?

The chief indication is the expectoration of solid chunks from the posterior nares, plugs or clinkers, so-called; in the morning lumps of green mucus are hawked from the posterior nares; the secretion is stringy and difficult to get out, there is dryness and tickling in the nose and sneezing, all worse in the open air.

Give indications for Kali carb.

Coryza, with hoarseness or loss of voice; catches cold

at every exposure to fresh air; stiff neck; elongated uvula; obstruction of nose relieved in open air, but returns on entering warm room.

What is the Catarrh of Aurum?

The nostrils are sore and cracked, the discharge is fetid and there is caries of the nasal bones; especially if of a scrofulous or mercurio-syphilitic origin.

How does Nitric acid compare here?

With *Nitric acid* there is ulceration and splinter-like pains in the naso-pharynx, the discharge is watery and offensive and very excoriating. Hard plugs in nose, which, when detached, leave a raw surface.

What are the indications for Hepar in colds?

Advanced stage when phlegm has formed with sticking in the throat; colds which are easily re-excited from any exposure.

What are the symptoms calling for Ammonium carb. in Catarrh?

The nose is stopped up and the patient is worse about three or four in the morning; the coryza is scalding and there is burning in the throat.

What is the Catarrh of Ammonium mur.?

There is stoppage of one nostril during the day and both at night; the coryza is scalding and the burning extends to the throat and trachea.

What are the symptoms of Bromine in Coryza?

Profuse, watery, excoriating discharge with headache and downward pressure at the root of the nose; the nose is very sore and smarts inside; ulcers form and scabs and crusts are blown out.

What are the nasal symptoms of Sambucus?

The nose is greatly stuffed up, and the child starts up as if suffocating; snuffles.

Give symptoms of Sticta.

Stuffed up nose; the secretion drying so rapidly that it cannot be discharged. Inclination to blow nose, but nothing escapes.

Give the indications for Arsenicum iodatum in Catarrhs.

Violent, acute coryza, with watery, acrid discharge, soreness in the nostrils, heat and burning extending into the eyes and headache.

What are the nasal symptoms of Lachesis?

Watery discharge, worse on the left side, with a throbbing headache, which is relieved when the discharge appears.

What are the characteristic indications for Verbascum?

Catarrhs and cold accompanied by neuralgia and a hoarse, barking cough, a sort of "*basso profundo.*" It also is a powerful remedy in urinary irritability. The preparation known as *Mullein oil* comes from the plant.

Give the symptoms of Cinnabaris in Nasal catarrh.

Pressure at the root of the nose, as if a heavy pair of spectacles were there; swollen and dry throat, with swollen tonsils, and stringy mucus in the posterior nares, which passes into the throat.

Give the symptoms of Wyethia, another useful remedy for Catarrhal troubles.

Dryness of pharynx with constant desire to clear throat; follicular pharyngitis, with a hot, burning feeling. Hoarseness, pharyngitis in teachers and singers.

What are some characteristic indications of Elaps in Catarrhal troubles?

Catarrhal snuffles in children, nose stuffed up; also the great sense of coldness that cold water leaves in the stomach.

Give an indication for Teucrium marum verum.

Catarrh, with expectoration of solid chunks from the posterior nares; nasal polypi.

Give the nasal symptoms of Sanguinaria.

Great susceptibility to odors, which causes the patient to faint; burning and rawness in the nose, with fluent coryza which excoriates; nasal polypi which tend to bleed easily.

What are the characteristic nasal symptoms of Phosphorus?

Caries of the bones of the nose; ulcerations of the nose with stoppage; hemorrhage and offensive odor; nasal polypi.

What are the Catarrhal symptoms of Natrum carb?

Fluent coryza, provoked by least draught of air, with a daily periodical aggravation; relieved by sweating. Chronic catarrh, ozæna, thick, yellowish discharge from nose, accumulation of mucus in posterior nares, causing hemming and hawking.

Give indications for Bryonia in Coryza.

Either great dryness or thick, yellowish discharge, especially when discharge has been suddenly suppressed and there is a throbbing headache in frontal sinuses.

How does Lachesis compare in suppressed coryza?

It is not aggravated by motion, nor has it the yellow discharge.

When is Rhus indicated?

Coryza, with severe aching in all the bones; sneezing and coughing from exposure to dampness.

How does Dulcamara compare?

Coryza, shivering, marked chilliness, sneezing and severe aching of long bones. Intermingling of heat and chill.

COLIC.

What is the greatest characteristic of Colocynth?

A violent, agonizing abdominal colic; relieved by bending double and by pressing something hard into the abdomen.

How does the Colic of Dioscorea differ from that of Colocynth?

The pains are apt to radiate from the abdomen to other parts of the body, as to back, arms, etc. It is relieved by walking and throwing the body backwards.

What other species of Colic is Colocynth useful for?

Ovarian colic; sharp pains in the ovarian regions, relieved by bending double and by pressure.

What is necessary for Colocynth to be of any use in any form of Colic?

That the nervous elements predominate over the inflammatory symptoms.

Give indications for Cuprum in Colic.

Knife-like, violent pains in the abdomen, which are better from pressure, but are not better from heat; there is neuralgia of all the abdominal nerves, as if a knife were drawn through to the back.

When should Magnesia phos. be used in Colic?

Where there is intense and spasmodic pain, forcing the patient to bend double, and accompanied by belching of gas, which does not relieve; the pains are greatly relieved by the application of warmth.

In what intestinal affection has Natrum sulphuricum also been found useful?

In lead colic.

What are the symptoms of Nux in Colic?

Flatulent colic with desire to stool, and a sensation as if the intestines were squeezed between stones.

What are the indications for the use of Plumbum in Lead Colic?

Horrible griping pain in the abdomen, with retraction of the abdominal walls; the pains radiate in all directions, following the course of the nerves.

Name some other remedies useful as antidotes to Lead Colic.

Nux vomica, Alumina, Platina, Opium, Alum and *Belladonna.*

Mention three drugs having Colic from a fit of anger.

Chamomilla, Staphisagria, and *Colocynth.*

Give the Colic of Ipecac.

Griping about umbilicus as of a hand clutching; cutting pains shooting across the abdomen, from left to right, associated with nausea and diarrhœa.

Give the indications for Veratrum.

Pains force patient to bend double; must walk about for relief; cold sweat on forehead.

CONSTIPATION.

What is the grand characteristic of the Bryonia Constipation?

When it is due to dryness of the intestinal tract and the stools are large, dry and brown, as if burnt, and are passed with a great deal of difficulty, owing to an atony of the intestines.

How does it differ from Nux vomica?

Nux vom. produces an increased intestinal action, which is irregular, inharmonious and spasmodic, and this hinders rather than favors an evacuation.

What other drugs besides Bryonia have Constipation with atony of the intestines?

Veratrum album and *Opium.*

To what is the Constipation of Opium due?

To complete inactivity of the bowels, owing to a muscular paresis. Under *Opium* the fæces become impacted and are passed in little, hard, dry, black balls, and there is absolutely no urging to stool.

How does Plumbum compare here?

Plumbum has stools consisting of hard, black balls, but there is some constriction of the rectum, showing that there is some activity of the muscles present.

What is the Constipation of Alumina?

There is complete inertia of the rectum, so that the stool is expelled with great difficulty, no matter what the consistency of it is; there is little or no urging to stool; the stools may be dry, hard and knotty, like sheep dung, or soft; constipation of children where the rectum is dry, hard, inflamed and bleeding.

To what is the Constipation of Alumina due?

Both to dryness and inactivity of the rectum, producing the symptom that soft stools are expelled with difficulty.

What is the stool of Anacardium?

There is a sensation of a plug in the rectum, it seems powerless to expel the stool; even a soft stool is expelled with difficulty.

What are the characteristic symptoms of Nux vom. in Constipation?

Inactivity, with constant, ineffectual urging to stool. The passages are incomplete and unsatisfactory, as if part remained behind.

How does Lycopodium compare here?

Lycopodium has ineffectual urging to stool, but under *Lycopodium* it is not due to irregular intestinal action, but to a constriction of the rectum.

How does Carbo veg. compare here?

Carbo veg. also has ineffectual urging to stool, but here it is due to flatulence.

How is Nux vom. distinguished from Opium, Bryonia and Alumina?

These drugs have no urging at all.

What are the symptoms of Lycopodium in Constipation?

Sensation as if something remained behind; constipation due to constriction of the rectum. It is a useful remedy in the constipation of young children; it is apt to be associated with hemorrhoids. There is a constricted feeling about the rectum, as in *Silicea*.

What is the remedy for Constipation due to abuse of purgative medicines?

Nux vomica.

What is the Constipation of Sulphur?

Ineffectual urging to stool with a sensation of heat, fulness and discomfort in the rectum. It is a useful remedy with which to commence the treatment of constipation. Uneasy feeling all through intestinal tract; constipation alternating with diarrhœa; abdominal plethora or passive portal congestion.

What is the characteristic indication for Graphites in Constipation?

It is where the stools are covered with mucus and there is no urging. The patient sometimes goes days without a stool, and when it does come it is composed of little round balls knotted together, with shreds of mucus and accompanied with great pain when passing, owing to fissure.

What is the Constipation of Platina?

Torpor of the whole intestinal tract; unsuccessful urging to stool and great dryness of the rectum. The stools adhere to the rectum like putty or glue. There is great weakness in the abdomen and a sensation as if there was a load in the rectum which could not be expelled. It is a remedy for the constipation of travelers and emigrants.

What is the Constipation of Natrum mur.?

The stools are hard and difficult to expel, causing bleeding and smarting and soreness in the rectum. There is dryness of the rectum and the stools are crumbly in character; great weakness of the intestine.

What is the characteristic Constipation of Phosphorus?

Where the stools are grayish, showing lack of bile. They are long, slender and tough, resembling a dog's stool, and voided with the utmost difficulty.

What is the great characteristic of Silicea in Constipation?

It is due to the deficient expulsive power of the rectum and spasmodic condition of the sphincter, which gives rise to the symptom that the stool slips back when partially expelled.

What symptoms has Ammonium muriaticum?

The stools are hard and crumbly, crumble as they pass the anus. All *Muriates* have crumbly stools.

Give the Constipation of Sepia.

No desire or urging for days and days; the stools are hard and large; inactivity of the rectum, and a sensation of a ball in it; patient cannot strain and consequently cannot expel stool.

What are the indications for Hydrastis in Constipation?

After the use of purgatives, when there is present the sinking, gone feeling at the epigastrium, and symptoms of gastro-duodenal catarrh, such as torpidity of the liver, yellow skin and tenderness in the hepatic region and light colored stools.

What is the constipation of Veratrum?

Large, hard black stools with faintness; patient strains until covered with cold sweat and then gives it up, and fæces accumulate in large masses in the rectum.

What are the characteristics of the Plumbum Constipation?

There is a marked retraction of the abdomen, and a spasm or contraction of the sphincter ani; there is urging to stool, and the stool is passed in little, round balls, which are black and hard; they are passed with great difficulty, and are often accompanied by colic or a sensation of a string pulling the anus up into the rectum.

What is peculiar about the stool of Causticum?

Owing to a paralytic condition of the rectum the patient is unable to evacuate the stool when sitting, he is obliged almost to stand.

When is Magnesia mur. indicated in Constipation?

Stools are passed with great difficulty, being composed of hard lumps, which are so dry that they crumble as they pass the anus.

What symptom has Selenium in common with Alumina, Opium, Plumbum and Bryonia?

The fæces are hard and dry and require artificial means for their removal. Peristaltic action is *nil* with this remedy.

CONVULSIONS.

What symptoms indicate Belladonna in Convulsions?

Convulsions following emotions; bright red face, hot head; child suddenly becomes rigid, stiffens out; foams at mouth; between them, startings from sleep, or deep moaning or crying out.

How does Cina compare?

Pale face, child stiffens out, restless; occurring as a result of irritation from worms or from dentition.

When is Chamomilla the remedy?

Convulsions after any emotion; child is petulant, one cheek is red the other pale; hot sweat about face and head.

When is Cocculus indicated in Spasms?

When due to irritable weakness, suppressed menses, loss of sleep.

What are the indications for Cuprum?

The fingers are clenched, blueness of face and mouth, and attempts to swallow fluids cause gurgling in throat.

What drugs have Convulsions with fingers spread asunder and extended?

Glonoine and *Secale*.

Give indications for Glonoine in Puerperal Convulsions.

Face bright red and puffed, pulse full; patient froths at mouth, is unconscious; congestive form, accompanied by rush of blood to head.

Give Convulsions of Hydrocyanic acid.

Lightning-like shocks pass through body; drawing at nape of neck; uræmic convulsions when medulla is affected; blue face, gasping breathing, clutching at heart and prostration.

When is Hyoscyamus indicated?

Sudden startling and twitching of the muscles, angular movements, frothing at mouth, wild look, biting of the tongue. Hunger before attacks.

How is Stramonium distinguished?

By its swollen, turgid face; by the renewal of the spasms by light, and the spasmodic actions are more graceful than angular.

Give symptoms calling for Ignatia.

Spasms brought on by emotions, as in children after punishment; twitching of muscles; child stiffens out.

How does Veratrum compare?

Also from emotions, but the face is cold and blue, and cold sweat covers the forehead.

What drug has Convulsions in children from over-indulgence in rich food?

Ipecac.

CORYZA.

(See Colds and Catarrh.)

COUGHS.

What is the Cough of Aconite?

The cough is hard, dry and barking. There is little or no expectoration.

Give the Cough of Aralia racemosa.

Spasmodic cough at night, coming on after the first sleep. Relief after expectoration of tough mucus.

Give Cough of Bromine.

Cough with much rattling on breathing. It seems as if the next cough would bring up a great quantity of mucus, but when the cough comes it is deep and hard.

What is the Cough of Bryonia?

It is caused by epigastric or supra-sternal irritation. The cough is dry, and the patient presses his hand against the sides to relieve the pain. It is a painful cough and hurts distant parts of the body, as for instance the head. It is worse in a warm room, and there is a slight yellowish or blood-streaked expectoration.

What is the Cough of Phosphorus?

There is a dry, tickling cough, which is worse from going from a warm room into the cold, or in changes from warm to cold caused by irritation in the larynx and beneath the sternum. There is a great deal of rawness in the larynx, and is worse from talking.

What is the Cough of Belladonna?

Cough from tickling in the larynx as from dust. Dry,

hacking cough coming on in violent attacks with an expectoration of blood-tinged mucus. Much pain in chest.

What is the Cough of Rumex crispus?

It is a teasing, persistent cough, aggravated by cold air. The patient has to put his head under the bed-clothes and breathe warm air to relieve the cough. It is caused by tickling in the supra-sternal fossa, and is worse at night from lying down. Night cough in phthisis.

What other drugs have a Cough worse at night on lying down?

Silicea, *Phosphorus* and *Lycopodium*.

What is the Cough of Drosera?

It is a spasmodic cough which comes on in the evening, and every effort to raise the phlegm ends in vomiting. In whooping cough the cough is so frequent that the patient cannot catch his breath. Must hold sides with hands.

What other drugs have this last symptom?

Eupatorium perf. and *Natrum sulph*.

What is the cough of Causticum?

There is a tickling cough which is relieved by a drink of cold water. There is often associated with the cough involuntary spurting of urine. There is a great deal of rawness in the throat and hoarseness and loss of voice.

What other drugs have involuntary spurting of urine during cough?

Squilla and *Natrum mur*.

What is the cough of Ignatia?

It is a nervous, dry spasmodic cough in quick, successive shocks, as if a feather were in the throat; the more the patient coughs the more he wants to, and it is only stopped by an effort of the will; the cough occurs in the evening on lying down.

What is the Cough of Kali bichromicum?

It is a hard, barking cough which seems to start from the epigastrium, and the expectoration is of a yellow, stringy character and difficult to raise.

How does Coccus cacti differ from Kali bich.?

Here the expectoration is ropy, but is clear albuminous mucus, and the remedy is especially indicated in whooping cough. The paroxyms of the cough end in vomiting of clear, ropy mucus which hangs in great long strings from the mouth.

Give Cough of Calcarea carb.

Cough excited by tickling as of a feather in the throat and with the cough a piercing pain in chest; cough dry at first, afterwards with profuse salty expectoration.

What is the Cough of Corallium rubrum?

It has been styled the "minute gun" cough, the paroxysms coming on very close together. It is a short, dry, ringing cough. It takes the child's breath away, so that when the paroxysms have ceased he feels exhausted.

What other drug has this symptom, and how does it differ?

Mephitis. It is indicated where the catarrhal symptoms are slight and the whoop is marked.

What is the Cough which calls for Hepar?

It is a hoarse, croupy cough, having withal a "loose edge," the phlegm being loose and choking; worse from exposure to cold air and from drinking cold water.

How is the Cough of Hepar distinguished from that of Belladonna, Conium, Rumex and Lachesis?

From *Belladonna* by absence of laryngeal soreness and fever.

From *Conium*, the irritation being higher in the throat.

From *Rumex* by not being affected by respiration.

From *Lachesis* by not being excited by pressure on larynx.

What is the Cough of Opium?

It has a dry, tickling cough, which is especially worse at night and is relieved by a drink of water.

Give the Cough of Conium.

Dry, spasmodic, hacking; worse at night upon lying down, and is fatiguing in old people; mucus cannot be expectorated, must be swallowed; the cough is caused by an irritation in the larynx as of a dry spot.

How does Hyoscyamus compare?

It lacks the dry spot of irritation of *Conium*

What is the Cough of Sticta?

Hard, dry, barking, almost croupy cough; worse at night with little or no expectoration. An irritable cough, caused by dryness high up in the pharynx; not aggravated by lying down, but worse at night.

Give the Cough of Squills.

Violent cough with a great deal of mucus in the chest and expectoration; during the cough there is involuntary spurting of urine; the patient coughs a long time before a little mucus is raised, which gives relief; sharp, sticking pains in side, which are worse during the cough.

What is the Cough of Hyoscyamus?

Cough which is aggravated lying down at night and relieved by sitting up; aggravated from eating, drinking and talking; cough from an elongated uvula.

How does Conium compare?

It has a cough at night aggravated by lying down; but it is caused by a dry spot sensation in the larynx, and the patient has to sit up.

What is there characteristic of the Cough of Cuprum?

It is relieved by a drink of cold water; cold water also relieves the vomiting; whooping cough, the attacks coming on in quick succession, relieved by a drink of water, accompanied perhaps by spasms, threatening suffocation.

What other drug has Cough relieved by a drink of water?

Causticum.

What are the indications for Laurocerasus in Cough?

Dry, teasing cough at night with expectoration tinged with blood; lack of reaction in chest troubles.

What is the Cough of Magnesia phosphorica?

True spasmodic cough, coming on in paroxysms, without expectoration. Whooping cough is worse at night and accompanied with difficulty in lying down.

What is the Cough of Nitric acid?

Dry, tickling cough, worse at night, and often starting from a particular spot in the larynx.

What is the Cough of Sepia?

Cough seeming to come from the stomach or abdomen; a cough with salty expectoration, attended by stitches in the epigastrium. Whooping cough with vomiting of bile and soreness of chest during cough; relieved by pressure.

Give a remedy sometimes useful in the dry, hacking Cough of consumptives.

Hydrocyanic acid.

What symptom has Eupatorium perf. that is similar to Bryonia?

The cough hurts head and chest; the patient holds the chest with the hands. Soreness in larynx, hoarseness and aching in loins.

What drug has a Cough that is worse when strangers are present?

Ambra grisea. It is purely a nervous cough.

What is the Cough of Kali sulph.?

Cough with great rattling of mucus on the chest, worse in a warm room, relieved in the cool, open air.

Give the Cough of Spongia.

Hard, ringing, metallic cough, worse from deep breathing, with a sensation of weakness. Better from warm drinks.

What is the Cough of Antimonium tart.?

The cough sounds loose, but no phlegm is raised; it seems as if every cough would raise the phlegm, but it does not. There is whistling and rattling extending into the trachea.

What is the Cough of Verbascum?

Hard, harsh and barking cough, with hoarseness; a tracheal and laryngeal cough.

CROUP.

When should Aconite be given?

When brought on by dry, cold winds; hard, dry, barking cough, heard all over the house. Difficult breathing, anxiety and fever.

What are indications for Bromine in Croup?

Deep, hoarse voice; inspiration produces coughing; the breathing is hoarse, rasping and whistling, and there is rattling in the larynx, and when the child coughs it sounds as if the larynx were full of mucus.

When is Iodine indicated in Croup?

It is very similar to *Bromine;* there is a hoarse voice and difficult inspiration; the child grasps at its throat; croup caused by long-continued damp weather, with more fever than in *Bromine*, and the general temperament of the drug.

What are the indications for Spongia in Croup?

The breathing is harsh and hard, as if the patient were breathing through a sponge; hard, barking, ringing cough with scanty expectoration; the cough seems to get tighter every minute; threatened suffocation.

When is Hepar the remedy?

When the cough is worse towards morning and there is rattling of mucus. Least exposure excites a fit of coughing. The cough begins to loosen, has a loose edge.

What are two remedies for Spasm of the Glottis?

Sambucus and *Chlorine*.

When is Antimonium tart. indicated in Croup?

When the rattling and wheezing extends down trachea; mucus râles, great prostration and dyspnœa.

Give indications for Kali bichromicum.

True membranous croup. Metallic sound to cough, labored breathing, rattling of mucus, smothering spells and characteristic stringy expectoration. Tendency to extend downward.

What other drug, not often used, is useful in Croup where the tendency of the disease is to extend to the trachea and upper chest?

Kaolin.

CYSTITIS.

(See Urinary Disorders.)

DEBILITY.

What is the great characteristic of Cinchona in cases of Debility?

Weakness, debility, and diseases resulting from the loss of vital fluids, such as blood, semen, milk, or in exhausting diarrhœas.

What is the Debility of Muriatic acid?

It is general and so great that the patient slips down to the foot of the bed and must be lifted up every little while; inability to void the urine unless the bowels move.

Describe the Debility calling for Phosphoric acid.

It is a nervous debility, arising from continued grief, over-exertion of mind, sexual excess or any nervous strain on the body; it is characterized by indifference, apathy, and torpidity of body and mind.

How does the Debility of Sulphuric acid show itself?

As a tremor; there is a sense of tremor accompanied by objective trembling; it is a debility which occurs at the change of life or in drunkards.

When is Arsenicum and Phosphorus indicated?

Arsenicum. Debility from overtaxing muscular tissues; mountain climbing.

Phosphorus. Nervous debility, with great drowsiness and sleepiness.

When, in debilitated conditions, is Cocculus the remedy?

When of spinal origin, from loss of sleep; where loss of sleep causes languor and exhaustion.

Give another drug having debility from loss of sleep.

Colchicum.

DELIRIUM.

What kind of a Delirium is produced by Absinthium?

Delirium with great desire to move about.

Give briefly the characteristic Delirium of Belladonna, Hyoscyamus and Stramonium, so that they may be distinguished.

Belladonna. Visions, screaming out and desire to escape, full of fear and imaginings, sensation as if falling, and the patient clutches the air; sometimes a stupor, when aroused they strike people, bark and bite like a dog and are very violent.

Hyoscyamus. Averse to light, fears being poisoned, sits up in bed and looks around, exposes sexual organs; is nervous, whining, crying and twitching.

Stramonium. Desires light and company; objects rise from every corner to frighten him; laughs, sings, swears and prays in the same breath; face bright red.

What is the Delirium of Phosphorus?

It is characterized by a condition of ecstasy; sees all sorts of faces grinning at him; has fanciful and imaginary notions, such as imagining his body in fragments.

Give Delirium of Veratrum.

Restless; desires to cut or tear clothing; in many respects like that of *Belladonna*, but there is coldness of the surface of the body, with cold sweat.

DELIRIUM TREMENS.

(See Alcoholism.)

DENTITION.

Give indications for Ferrum phos.

Feverishness, flushed face, sparkling eyes, dilated pupils; restlessness and irritability.

When is Calcarea phosphorica indicated in Dentition?

There is slow development and rapid decay of the teeth, dental troubles in flabby, emaciated children who have open posterior fontanelles, and are slow in learning to walk.

When is Chamomilla the remedy?

The characteristic mental state of peevishness is present; one cheek is red, head and scalp hot and sweaty.

How does Belladonna compare?

In further advanced cases where there is evidence of cerebral irritation with the characteristic generalities of the drug; spasms.

When is Kreosote indicated?

Child worries and must be tossed and patted all night; teeth decay rapidly.

DIABETES.

Give some indications for Arsenicum.

Unquenchable thirst and great hunger; dryness of mouth, excessive urination and loss of strength.

Give the indications for Phosphoric acid in Diabetes.

Glycosuria and *Polyuria;* urine looks milky or like jelly after standing; great debility; cough on slightest exposure; bruised feeling in muscles and burning in the spine; urine loaded with phosphates showing a greasy pellicle.

What are some clinical indications for Uranium nitricum, another remedy for Diabetes?

Emaciation, excessive thirst, vomiting of food with excessive urine; sometimes tympanites.

Mention another remedy having a reputation for usefulness in Diabetes.

Lactic acid.

DIARRHŒA.

When is Aconite indicated in Diarrhœa?

When of inflammatory origin with watery, slimy and bloody stools; occurring in summer from cold drinks or checked perspiration; also chopped spinach stools.

Give Diarrhœa of Aloes.

Stools of jelly-like mucus, a weak sphincter ani, with great prostration following; the patient loses confidence in his sphincter and passes stools when he thinks he is passing wind; stools are involuntary. There is a weight and fulness in the pelvic region. This full feeling drives patient out of bed in morning for stool.

How is this compared with the Diarrhœa of Apocynum can.?

Here we have a copious yellow or watery diarrhœa discharged with force, like a cork from a bottle; stools escape while passing flatus, and after stool an all gone feeling in abdomen.

What drug has a stool expelled all at once, preceded by cutting about navel, followed by great relief?

Gamboge.

Give Diarrhœa of Apis.

Thin, watery, yellow diarrhœa, worse in the morning, in debilitated children. The bowels move with every motion of the body as if the anus stood open.

What other drug has the symptom of a sensation as if the anus stood open?

Phosphorus, which has green mucous stools worse in the morning, often undigested and painless. The stools pass as soon as they enter the rectum; contain white particles like rice or tallow.

Give Diarrhœa of Argentum nitricum.

Diarrhœa following great excitement, fright, etc. The stools are slimy and green with much flatulence, worse at night. The bowels move every time the patient drinks; the child appears to have but one bowel extending from mouth to anus.

What other drugs have Diarrhœa from fright?

Gelsemium, *Opium*, *Veratrum alb.* and *Pulsatilla*.

What drug has Diarrhœa as soon as the patient attempts to eat?

Ferrum met.

What drugs have Diarrhœa after eating?

China and *Arsenicum*.

What is the Diarrhœa of Arnica?

The stools are foul, slimy, bloody and even purulent; there is great urging and straining.

Give in brief the indications for Arsenicum in Diarrhœa.

The stools are yellow, undigested, slimy or bloody; they are scanty and attended with great burning in the rectum, the burning being all out of proportion to the stools. These are the characteristics:
1. The small quantity.
2. The burning.
3. The offensive odor.
4. The great prostration following.

Compare Carbo veg. with Arsenicum.

Also a useful remedy for diarrhœa from chilling of the stomach, but has no restlessness.

How does Secale compare?

The Secale movements are copious and come in spurts, with no restlessness.

HOMŒOPATHIC THERAPEUTICS.   65

Give the stool of Mercurius.

The stools are slimy and bloody and accompanied by great tenesmus, which continues after stool, "a never get done feeling."

Is Belladonna ever indicated in Diarrhœa?

When it arises from cold and is associated with tenesmus, with slimy and bloody discharges; stools may be yellowish green, looking like chalk; summer complaints of children.

What is the stool of Chamomilla?

Hot, yellowish-green diarrhœa like chopped eggs, mixed with bile and causing soreness of the anus, and having a sulphuretted-hydrogen odor; worse evenings and from dentition.

What other drug has a hot stool smelling like rotten eggs?

Staphisagria.

Name some remedies having greenish stools.

Borax, Calc. phos., Magnes. carb. and *Hepar*.

Give the Diarrhœa of Hepar.

Greenish, slimy, undigested, white or sour; the whole child smells sour.

Name four prominent remedies for sour stools.

Magnes. carb., Calcarea carb., Hepar and *Rheum*.

What are the symptoms calling for Rheum?

Sour stools, the whole body smells sour; stools are frequent, brown and frothy, attended with straining and crying.

How does Magnesia carb. differ here?

Both have sour, slimy stools. *Magnesia* is the deeper acting remedy.

What is the Diarrhœa of Bryonia?

It is a morning diarrhœa, worse from motion, provoked by indulgence in vegetable foods or stewed fruit or by getting overheated; it comes on after getting up and moving about; stools are pasty or dark green; involuntary discharge of thin stool while sleeping at night.

What other drug has a morning Diarrhœa which is worse after getting up and moving about?

Natrum sulph.

Mention some other drugs which have early morning Diarrhœa.

Sulphur, Kali bi., Aloes and *Rumex*.

What is the Diarrhœa of Sulphur?

The stools are changeable in color and may contain undigested food. It occurs in the morning and drives the patient out of bed; there is a great deal of abdominal uneasiness; the odor of the stool clings to the patient for a long time, and there is much soreness at the anus.

How does the stool of Podophyllum compare?

It has a morning stool, with a great deal of soreness and fullness in the region of the liver, and it continues throughout the day.

How is Rumex distinguished?

It has a morning diarrhœa associated with catarrhs.

What is the stool of Kali bich.?

It is a watery, gushing stool, with urging and tenesmus; he has not time to reach the closet and stains the bed-clothes.

Mention three prominent drugs having undigested stools.

China, *Podophyllum* and *Ferrum*.

What is the Diarrhœa of China?

Evacuations are watery and contain undigested food; the stools are debilitating and may be involuntary; worse after eating fruit; stools may be yellow, watery, brown and offensive; worse after eating; is usually painless.

How is Phosphoric acid differentiated?

The *Phosphoric acid* diarrhœa does not exhaust; otherwise it is similar to *China*. It is also painless.

Give Diarrhœa of Calcarea acetica.

It is exactly the same as that of *Phosphoric acid* with the addition of the general symptoms of *Calcarea* and sourness of stools.

What is the Diarrhœa of Oleander?

Thin, undigested stools, the patient passing what he had eaten the day before, undigested. In children "every time they pass wind they soil the diapers."

Give the Ferrum Diarrhœa.

Painless, undigested stool, apt to occur during a meal. It may occur quite periodically after midnight Great hunger. Eating brings on diarrhœa.

Give the characteristics of Podophyllum in Diarrhœa.

A painless morning diarrhœa of watery, yellow stools, which are profuse and pour out like water from a hydrant, preceded by retching and vomiting followed by a sensation of great weakness in the abdomen, and especially in the rectum; the stools are worse after eating and drinking, and there is apt to be a natural stool later in the day.

Is it ever useful in the Diarrhœas of dentition?

In greenish, watery stools, with grinding of the teeth, rolling of the head, with whining and moaning during sleep, it is an excellent remedy.

What is another indicating feature of Podophyllum in Diarrhœa?

Prolapsus of the rectum during stool.

What drug has profuse, watery, yellowish-green discharges whenever the patient eats or drinks, gushing out like water from a hydrant?

Croton tig.

What other drug has a like symptom and what is its characteristic feature?

Gratiola, and it is caused by excessive drinking of water, especially in summer.

What is the Diarrhœa of Elaterium?

Watery, frothy diarrhœas with copious, forcible stools, preceded by violent cutting in the abdomen, chilliness, prostration and colic; olive green stools, but always gushing.

Give four grand characteristics of the stool of Veratrum.

1. Pain in abdomen preceding stool.
2. Cold sweat accompanying.
3. Great prostration following.
4. Profuse, watery discharges.

What is the stool of Jatropha?

Violent, watery stool, preceded by much flatulence, with prostration and collapse. The excessive flatulence is the indicating feature. It is discharged with the stool.

When is Colocynth indicated in Diarrhœa?

Stools are preceded by griping in the abdomen and are provoked by the slightest food or drink. The stools are fluid, copious or papescent and the griping is relieved by bending double.

What is the Diarrhœa of Dioscorea?

Morning diarrhœa with colicky pains in the abdomen, which, however, are apt to fly to other parts of the body.

Mention a few not often used remedies which should be borne in mind in cases of Diarrhœa.

Œnothera biennis, Gnaphalium, Geranium mac., Paullinia sorbilis, Nuphar luteum, Kali bromatum and *Opuntia*.

Give the Stool of Iris versicolor.

Copious stools associated with vomiting; worse at two or three o'clock in the morning; there is no coldness or collapse; excoriated feeling about anus; stools watery, yellowish-green, mixed with bile.

Give Diarrhœa of Petroleum

Offensive, watery stools, containing undigested food, comes on in morning and lasts all day. Diarrhœa from cabbage or sauer kraut; there is also emaciation.

When is Pulsatilla indicated in Diarrhœa?

Greenish stools, yellowish and changeable, occurring often after fright or after taking mixed food the night before; eating ice cream, immediately after a meal.

What is the Diarrhœa of Ipecac?

Green, yellow, liquid stools covered with mucus and blood or fermented and looking like molasses, associated with colic.

What remedy has a suddenly appearing Diarrhœa from fright or excitement?

Gelsemium.

What are the characteristics of the Diarrhœa of Leptandra?

Black, pitch-like stools, with colic at the umbilicus.

When is Lachesis indicated in Diarrhœa?

Horribly offensive diarrhœa, preceded by sopor; the offensiveness of the stool indicates it in low forms of disease; constant urging in the rectum and a sensation as of little hammers there; the sphincter is unduly irritable.

What are the Stools of Nitric acid?

Offensive, greenish, and contain lumps of casein; slimy and associated with tenesmus and soreness about anus. There may be pasty and sour stools, particularly in scrofulous children.

What drug is indicated in Diarrhœa from drinking Cocoa or Chocolate?

Lithium carb.

When is Nux vomica indicated in Diarrhœas?

When they occur after a debauch and are worse in the morning; they are papescent, scanty and watery, and accompanied by urging.

What are the symptoms calling for Rhus tox?

A bloody, slimy diarrhœa, or an involuntary stool of cadaverous odor in typhoid fever.

Give five drugs which have especially offensive Stools

Carbo veg., *Silicea*, *Psorinum*, *Sulphur* and *Podophyllum*.

What is the Diarrhœa of Ferrum phos.?

Undigested, copious and sudden, may be watery or greenish mucus; diarrhœa during dentition.

Give indications for Natrum phos. in Diarrhœa.

Sour smelling, greenish stools; mucus with painful straining, excoriating parts as they pass.

What is there characteristic of the Stools of Hyoscyamus?

They are involuntary in low delirious conditions.

What is the Stool of Chelidonium?

It is a bright yellow or clayey diarrhœa.

How does Mercurius differ?

It has the hepatic soreness and tongue taking the imprints of the teeth, but it also has slimy stools, with a great deal of tenesmus—a never-get-done feeling.

What is the Diarrhœa of Calcarea phosphorica?

Diarrhœa in teething, scrofulous and rachitic children; the stools are green, slimy and undigested; it is a noisy, offensive, watery and *spluttering* diarrhœa; cholera infantum, with a great deal of offensive flatus.

What is the Diarrhœa of Carbo vegetabilis?

Thin, watery, morning diarrhœa, accompanied by straining and urging to stool, which is due to flatulence; the discharges are offensive and burn the parts.

Give the Diarrhœa of Phosphoric acid.

It is a watery, painless, oftentimes undigested, diarrhœa, preceded by rumbling in the bowels, and despite the frequency of the stool the patient does not seem weakened by it; the keynotes are absence of pain and absence of exhaustion.

Give also the Diarrhœa of Euphorbia corrollata.

Diarrhœa, with vomiting, purging, and cold sweat over the body.

What is the Diarrhœa of Thuja?

Chronic diarrhœa traceable to vaccination, forcibly expelled like water from a bunghole; thirst with same gurgling sound on drinking, worse in the morning after breakfast, from coffee and onions, with rapid emaciation and exhaustion.

Give the Diarrhœa of Natrum muriaticum.

It is a diarrhœa which is watery and accompanied with great weakness of the abdominal muscles, and is sometimes involuntary.

What is the Diarrhœa of Dulcamara?

Yellow, watery diarrhœa in damp weather, or in summer, when the weather suddenly cools; mucous, green or changeable stools of sour odor. Diarrhœa from repelled eruptions.

What are the Stool symptoms of Colchicum?

Abdomen is distended enormously, with urging to stool and passage of jelly-like mucus; there are also dysenteric symptoms, with spasm of the sphincter ani.

DIPHTHERIA.

Give the symptoms calling for Apis in Diphtheria.

Great œdema of the throat; stinging pains; elongated, swollen and œdematous uvula and tonsils; breathing is difficult from swelling of the throat and tongue; the throat has a red, varnished appearance.

When would Arsenicum be indicated in Diphtheria?

Where there is adynamic fever, fetid breath, and the membrane looks dark and gangrenous, where the pulse is rapid and weak; the patient restless and prostrated, with throat swollen both externally and internally, and the membrane has a dark and wrinkled appearance, and where there is considerable œdema about the throat.

Give four indications for the use of Kali bichromicum in Diphtheria.

1. Yellow-coated or dry, red tongue.
2. In the later stage, when the line of demarcation has formed and the slough has commenced to separate.
3. Tough, tenacious exudation.
4. Pain extending to neck and shoulders.

Give indications for Kali permanganicum in Diphtheria.

Throat swollen inside and outside; the membrane is horribly offensive; throat œdematous, thin discharge from nose; fetor is the characteristic.

What are the indications for Lac caninum in Diphtheria?

Where the membrane forms on one side and goes to the other, or is constantly changing sides; the membrane is mother-of-pearl like.

What are the indications for Lachesis in Diphtheria?

Great difficulty in swallowing, great fetor and exhaustion, infiltration of tissues about the neck, membrane more on left side. Great sensitiveness of throat externally. Throat worse from empty swallowing.

Give indications for Mercurius cyanatus in Diphtheria.

Malignant type of diphtheria, with extreme prostration; where the disease invades the nostrils and there is a formation of membrane, which is at first white, then dark and gangrenous; the breath is fetid, the tongue is coated, and nosebleed is often present.

When are other varieties of Mercury indicated?

Merc. bin. iod. Membrane on left side, yellowish-gray in color. Glands of neck swollen. Symptoms worse from empty swallowing.

Merc. prot. Deposit on right side; glands swollen. Thick, yellow, dirty coating at base of tongue. Much tenacious mucus in throat.

When is Ailanthus the remedy in Diphtheria and when Arum triphyllum?

They both have excoriating discharges from the mouth and nose; they both have swellings of the throat inside and out, but *Ailanthus* is drowsy, lies in a stupor and is torpid, while *Arum* has restless tossing about.

What of Alcohol in this disease?

It tends to counteract the terrible prostration as well as to destroy the diphtheritic growth.

When is Baptisia useful?

When the disease assumes a typhoid type. The mouth

is putrid and the membrane dark and gangrenous. The patient can only swallow liquids.

When, if ever, should Bromine be given?

In the laryngeal form, with much rattling in the larynx; of most use in the croupoid form.

What are the indications for Lycopodium?

The right side is most affected, and the disease travels towards the left. The nose is stuffed up; constant desire to swallow, with stinging pains; patient is worse from 4 to 8 P. M.

When is Muriatic acid indicated in Diphtheria?

Malignant cases, with intense prostration; breath fetid; uvula œdematous. Discharges very excoriating.

When is Nitric acid to be thought of?

When the disease progresses and affects the stomach. Nasal diphtheria. Discharge watery, offensive, excoriating; sensation of splinter in throat, fetid odor, intermittent pulse.

What is the characteristic of Phytolacca?

The muscular aching, the dark red purple look and the aggravation from hot drinks.

Why should not local applications be used in this disease?

Because it is not a local, but a constitutional disease.

DROPSICAL AFFECTIONS.

What are our principal uses of Acetic acid?

In dropsies, standing midway between *Arsenic* and *Apis*,

distinguished from both in the characteristic thirst, and the predominance of the gastric symptoms.

Give the symptoms of Apis in Dropsy.

The skin is waxy and transparent like alabaster; the urine is scanty and albuminous, or with a dark sediment like coffee grounds. Absence of thirst, bruised feeling of abdominal walls, stinging pains, urine scanty, etc.

How does Acetic acid compare here?

There is a waxy look about the face and limbs and a great predominance of gastric symptoms, thirst and waterbrash.

What is the chief Homœopathic use of Apocynum can.?

In dropsical conditions, such as hydrocephalus and abdominal dropsies, where it is given as a diuretic; the principal indication is a copious yellow or brownish diarrhœa, expelled with great force, and a weak, all-gone feeling in the abdomen; oppression about the epigastrium and chest. Irritable stomach, drinking causes distress, though thirst is great. Dropsy, especially from liver affections.

How does it differ from Arsenic and from Apis?

It has unquenchable thirst. *Arsenic* wants little and often, *Apis* thirstless. The bloating in *Apocynum* is on the side on which he lies. *Arsenic* in the extremities. *Apis* under the eyes.

What are the indications for Digitalis in Dropsies?

Dropsies from cardiac affections; urine scanty, dark, hot; infiltration of scrotum and penis. Feeble pulse, feeling as if the heart stood still; constant desire to take a deep breath. Post-scarlatinal nephritis.

What are the indications for Lachesis?

The urine is dark and contains albumen, and the skin covering the œdematous parts is dark, bluish black.

When is Arsenic indicated?

In all forms of dropsy; transparent, waxy skin, intolerable thirst, spells of suffocation, worse at night, great dyspnœa.

Give symptoms calling for Lycopodium.

Dropsies of lower half of body from liver disease; legs swollen and covered with ulcers, from which serum oozes.

DYSENTERY.

When is Aconite the remedy in Dysentery?

Especially when it occurs in the autumn, when the days are warm and the nights are cold; stool frequent, scanty and with tenesmus. Hot, dry skin and general *Aconite* symptoms.

What are the indications for Capsicum in Dysentery?

Stools small and frequent; slimy; with burning and tenesmus, with thirst, yet drinking causes shivering. Soreness of anus.

What are the indications for Aloes in Dysentery?

The stools are of a jelly-like mucus and covered with blood, accompanied by griping in the epigastric region.

What are the indications for Arsenicum in Dysentery?

Scanty stools, burning in the rectum; tenesmus and thirst, and great prostration following.

What are the symptoms of Cantharis in Dysentery?

Discharge of blood-streaked mucus, looking like scraping of the intestines; cutting and burning in the anus; the tenesmus of the bladder predominates over that of the intestines.

What remedy clinically has proved useful in Dysentery?

Ferrum phos. In cases which are less acute than those calling for *Aconite*. There is more blood also with the stool. All the symptoms are less intense than those calling for *Aconite*.

When is Mercurius corrosivus indicated in Dysentery?

When the tenesmus is extreme, and when the stools are scanty, of mucus and blood, with great burning at the anus, and at the same time tenesmus of the bladder.

Compare Carbo veg. and Cinchona in Dysentery.

Both have dark, offensive, fluid discharges; both have distension of stomach; both have great weakness and hippocratic face. *Cinchona* alone has movement provoked by eating. The flatus of *Carbo veg.* is much more offensive.

Give a differentiating point between Mercurius and Nux vomica.

In *Nux vomica* the desire ceases after stool; in *Mercurius* it continues.

DYSMENORRHŒA.

When is Belladonna the remedy in painful menstruation?

There is pain preceding flow, and a sensation as if

everything would protrude from the vulva, relieved by sitting up straight; pains come on suddenly and cease suddenly; offensive clotted flow; congestive form of dysmenorrhœa.

When should Cactus be thought of?

Menses scanty and too early; cease when lying down; pain recurs periodically.

What are the indications for Cimicifuga in this affection?

Severe pains in back and down thighs, cramps and tenderness across hypogastrium; rheumatic, irritable uterus. The pains are neuralgic in character and bearing down. Often, hysterical symptoms accompany.

How does Caulophyllum compare?

Spasmodic dysmenorrhœa, bearing down pains, scanty flow; it produces a continued spasm of the uterus.

Give indications for Pulsatilla.

The menstrual flow comes by fits and starts, griping pains doubling patient up; patient tosses about and cries on account of pain.

What are the indications calling for Chamomilla?

Discharge dark and clotted, with tearing pains, excessive irritability and impatience.

When should Viburnum be chosen?

In spasmodic dysmenorrhœa with severe pain in lower part of abdomen, preceding flow.

Give indications for Magnesia phos.

Crampy neuralgic pains preceding the flow several hours; continue during flow. Warmth is grateful, and motion aggravates. Said to be useful in membranous Dysmenorrhœa.

What other Drugs are useful in membranous Dysmenorrhœa?

Borax and *Caulophyllum*.

Mention another remedy useful in neuralgic Dysmenorrhœa with pains extending down thighs.

Xanthoxylum.

DYSPEPSIA.

(See Gastric Derangements.)

EARS, DISEASES OF.

Give the ear symptoms of Belladonna.

Severe boring pains in the ears, which come on suddenly and shoot from one ear into the other.

What are the ear symptoms of Causticum?

Words, sounds and the patient's own voice re-echo in the ears; roaring and rushing noises in the ears.

Give five indications for Ferrum phosphoricum in ear troubles.

1. Diffused inflammatory processes.
2. Dark beefy redness of parts.
3. Muco-purulent discharge with tendency to hemorrhage.

4. The complete establishment of the discharge is not followed by relief of pain.

5. The paroxysmal character of the pain.

Give the ear symptoms of Kali muriaticum.

Deafness from swelling of the Eustachian tubes; proliferous catarrhal inflammation of the middle ear with thickening of the membrane; there is a stuffy sensation and obstruction of the naso-pharynx with snapping noises in the ear; also in deafness from swelling of the external ear.

Give some characteristic ear symptoms of Lachesis.

Roaring and singing in the ears, which is relieved by putting the finger in the ear and shaking it. Ears full of pasty, offensive wax.

What are the ear symptoms of Phosphorus?

Hardness of hearing and a re-echoing of sounds in the ears.

What are the ear symptoms of Psorinum?

Ottorrhœa, with a horribly offensive odor, like that of rotten meat.

What are the symptoms calling for Pulsatilla in Earache?

Sharp, tearing and pulsating pains, which are worse at night; earache in children.

When should Chamomilla be given instead?

In nervous children who cannot tolerate pain, and where one cheek is red and the other pale.

Mention two other remedies useful in Earache?

Dulcamara and *Borax*.

What are the ear symptoms of Silicea?

It is a useful remedy in suppurative ear troubles, accompanied by caries in the mastoid cells.

Mention another remedy useful for Earache when suppuration impends.

Hepar.

What drugs especially affect the mastoid process, producing Caries?

Aurum, Nitr. ac., Capsicum, Hepar, Silicea and *Carbo an.*

Give ear symptoms of Graphites.

The ears are too dry; hardness of hearing; better from riding in a carriage. Cracking in ears when swallowing or chewing.

ECZEMA.

(See Skin, Diseases of.)

ENURESIS.

(See Urinary Disorders.)

EPILEPSY.

What is the chief sphere of action of Cicuta virosa?

In spasms, with rigidity, fixed, staring eyes, blue face and frothing at the mouth; there is great difficulty in breathing, opisthotonos and loss of consciousness, and these spasms are followed by profound exhaustion.

What are the indications for Cuprum in Spasms?

When from suppressed eruptions; violent delirium, there is blueness of the face and lips, the eyeballs are distorted, and there is frothing at the mouth, and they may be ushered in by a shriek or cry. Convulsions following cholera.

Give the principal Homœopathic indications for Hydrocyanic acid.

In convulsions simulating epilepsy, tetanus with stiffness about the jaws and neck; another symptom indicating its use is a gurgling, which extends from the throat to the stomach when swallowing.

What are the convulsive symptoms of Hyoscyamus?

Epileptic spasms with jerking, twitching and frothing at the mouth, followed by sleep; patient bites his tongue; patient looks wild.

What do we use Œnanthe crocata for?

It has been used with success in epilepsy and paralytic conditions; convulsions with death-like syncope.

What is the characteristic of Silicea in Epilepsy?

Epilepsy which occurs at night, the aura beginning in the solar plexus; arising from overstrain of the mind and from emotion.

What are the symptoms of Artemisia in Epilepsy?

In cases which have arisen from fright.

If Epilepsy is caused by indigestion, the aura starting in the epigastrium and spreading upward, what is the remedy?

Nux vomica.

Mention a useful remedy for the attacks.

Hyoscyamus.

What drugs have Epilepsy with aura beginning in the solar plexus and proceeding upward?

Nux vomica, Silicea, Bufo and *Calcarea carb.*

What are useful remedies for Epilepsy and spasms which are caused from irritation of worms?

Indigo and *Cina.*

What is the character of the Bufo Epilepsy?

The aura starts from the epigastrium and from the genital organs. There is often preceding the attack great irritability of mind.

Give symptoms indicating Argentum nitricum.

Epilepsy from fright or coming on during menstruation; pupils are dilated for days or hours before attack; after attack restlessness and trembling of hands.

When is Cicuta virosa the remedy?

When the patient is taken with rigidity, fixed, staring eyes, blue face, frothing at mouth; shocks or series of shocks pass through body; jaws locked; followed by profound exhaustion.

EPISTAXIS.

(See Hemorrhages.)

ERYSIPELAS.

Give the symptoms of Apis in Erysipelas.

It is of a rosy, pinkish hue, later livid and purple, the parts become quickly œdematous, and there is a bruised, sore feeling to the skin.

What is the Erysipelas of Belladonna?

Bright red, rapid swelling of the skin, the skin is smooth, shining and tense; the pains are sharp, lancinating, stinging and throbbing.

How does Lachesis compare here?

The face is purplish instead of red, and the patient is drowsy and weaker.

What are the indications for Cantharis in facial Erysipelas.

Erysipelas beginning on the dorsum of the nose and spreading to the right cheek with the formation of large vesicles, which break and discharge an excoriating fluid.

Give indications for Euphorbium off. in Erysipelas.

In the vesicular form, where there are large, yellow vesicles and violent fever; pains extend from gums into ear.

Give the indications for Lachesis in facial Erysipelas.

More on the left side, at first bright red then dark bluish or purplish, great infiltration of cellular tissues and great weakness; patient drowsy and perhaps has delirium and is loquacious.

What variety of Erysipelas does Rhus correspond to?

The vesicular variety, where the skin looks dark and is covered with vesicles.

When is Stramonium indicated in Erysipelas?

When there are brain complications, such as violent delirium, screaming out, terrified.

EYE, DISEASES OF.

What are the characteristic eye symptoms of Apis?

Asthenopia and chemosis, a puffiness of the conjunctiva showing œdema. Œdematous swelling of the lids and especially below the eyes.

How does Apis compare with Rhus in eye affections?

There is less tendency to formation of pus with *Apis* than with *Rhus*. *Rhus* is relieved by warmth and *Apis* by cold.

What are the eye symptoms of Argentum nitr.?

Violent, purulent ophthalmia, with thick, yellow, bland discharge; the characteristic is the profuseness of the discharge.

Give the eye symptoms of Aurum.

Syphilitic iritis after the abuse of *Mercury;* ulceration of the cornea and intense photophobia; double vision and half vision, in which the lower half of objects can be seen.

What are the eye symptoms of Belladonna?

Sudden pains and violent symptoms, eyes feel swollen and protruding, conjunctiva red and pupils very much dilated, eyes feel as if full of sand, desire to rub the eyes which relieves. Great photophobia.

Give the eye symptoms of Causticum.

There is paralysis of the eyelids; there is heat, burning and feeling of sand in the eyes, muscular weakness and double vision.

What peculiar eye symptom has Cantharis?

Objects look yellow.

What are the eye symptoms of Cinnabaris?

A pain in the eye, which starts from one canthus and goes around the brow of the eye to the other canthus, a ciliary neuralgia.

What drug has a pain in the right eye as if it were pushed out of the head, worse near a warm stove?

Comocladia dentata.

Give eye symptoms of Euphrasia.

Blepharitis, injected eyes, discharge thick and excoriating, the tears scald and irritate the cheeks, photophobia worse in artificial light. Traumatic conjunctivitis. Paralysis of the third nerve.

How is Allium cepa distinguished?

The discharge from the eye in *Euphrasia* is excoriating and that from the nose is bland, while the opposite is found in *Allium cepa*, nose excoriating and eyes bland.

Give the eye symptoms of Ferrum phosphoricum.

Eyes inflamed, red, with a sensation as if grains of sand were under the lids; pain on moving the eyes; photophobia worse from artificial lights.

How does Gelsemium dilate the pupils?

By paralyzing the third nerve, which supplies the circular fibres of the iris; there being no longer any resistance to the action of the radiating fibres, the pupil dilates.

How does Belladonna dilate the pupil?

By stimulating the sympathetic, which supplies the radiating fibres of the iris, so that they overcome the action of the circular fibres.

When will Physostigma contract the pupils?

As this drug contracts the pupil by stimulating the third nerve, it will only contract the pupil dilated by the action of *Belladonna*, and not that dilated by the action of *Gelsemium*.

What are some other eye symptoms of Gelsemium?

It causes paralytic symptoms, such as diplopia or double vision from paresis of the eye muscles. Ptosis and strabismus; all from its action on the third nerve.

What are the eye symptoms of Graphites?

There is inflammation about the lids, which is especially worse about the canthi. There is a tendency for the edges of the lids to crack and bleed, styes appear, the lashes turn in, and there is a discharge from the eyes, which excoriates, and there are often vesicles on the cornea.

What are the eye symptoms of Hepar?

Purulent affections about the eyes, hypopyon, etc.; worse from cold air or cold applications.

In what affection of the eye is Kali bich. the remedy?

Ulcers of the cornea, with tendency to deep perforation; look as if punched out.

What are the characteristic eye symptoms of Kali muriaticum?

Parenchymatous keratitis and ulcerations of a low type where the redness of the conjunctiva is not excessive; photophobia, pain and lachrymation are moderate or absent, the base of the ulcer is dirty yellow, and the discharge is white mucus, and it tends to spread from the periphery.

Give the eye symptoms of Kali sulphuricum.

In ophthalmias where there is a profuse discharge of pus; ophthalmia neonatorum, crusts on the eyelids.

Give three characteristic symptoms of Mercurius in the eyes.

1. Muco-purulent discharges, which cause soreness of the lids and ulceration.
2. Sensitiveness and soreness of eyes to touch, with burning.
3. Intolerance of eyes to firelight, with dimness of vision.

Give the eye symptoms of Mercurius corrosivus.

Burning pains; intense photophobia and excoriating lachrymation, making the cheeks sore, almost taking the skin off; tearing in the bones around the eye; ulceration of cornea with tendency to perforation; it is almost specific for syphilitic iritis.

What are the characteristic eye symptoms of Natrum mur.?

It is a remedy especially characteristic in muscular asthenopia and in ciliary neuralgia, which comes and goes with the sun. Also in blepharitis. There is lachrymation and scalding, and letters run together when reading

What are the eye symptoms of Paris quadrifolia?

Sensation as if the eyes were drawn back into the head by strings.

What two conditions about the eye is Phosphorus useful in?

1. Cataract, the letters appear red; early in the disease.
2. Degeneration, or gray atrophy of the optic nerve from overwrought nervous system; objects have a cloudiness about them by candle light; green halo about objects.

What is the remedy for Atrophy of the optic nerve from tobacco?

Arsenicum.

Give eye symptoms of Rhus tox.

Conjunctivitis and iritis, when of traumatic or rheumatic origin, with severe pains worse at night; scrofulous ophthalmia and orbital cellulitis; ptosis and stiffness of the lids in rheumatic subjects. Œdematous swelling and acrid discharge.

What other drugs have this stiffness of the lids?

Causticum, *Gelsemium* and *Kalmia*.

What are the chief eye symptoms of Staphisagria which have been verified clinically?

Itching of margin of lids, styes, nodosities, chalazæ on lids, one after another, sometimes ulcerating.

Give some other drugs useful in Styes.

Pulsatilla, *Lycopodium* and *Hepar*.

What eye affections indicate Silicea?

Styes or pustular affections about the eyes.

In what affections about the eye is Spigelia useful?

Ciliary-neuralgia, pains radiate, cold feeling in the eye.

What other drug has cold feeling in the eye?

Thuja.

What are the eye indications for Pulsatilla?

Conjunctivitis; discharge thick, yellow and bland; ophthalmia after measles; ophthalmia neonatorum.

When would Zincum be indicated?

Opacities of cornea; pterygium; granular lids; amblyopia accompanied by headache with pain at root of nose; pains worse at inner canthus.

When is Ruta indicated in eye troubles?

When there is irritability of every tissue of the eye from overwork, such as using eyes on too fine work. Asthenopia, burning in the eyeballs and over the eyes, blurring of vision, letters seem to run together.

Give two remedies similar.

Belladonna and *Ammoniac gum.*

When is Aconite indicated in Conjunctivitis?

When resulting from a foreign body in the eye, or from exposure to dry, cold winds, there is heat, burning and a feeling of sand in the eyes. Much photophobia and violent aching in eyeballs, also in glaucoma.

When Aconite fails in Conjunctivitis resulting from a foreign body what is the remedy?

Sulphur.

Give the eye symptoms of Arsenicum.

Burning in the eyes like fire; phlyctenulæ on cornea; excoriating discharge from eye.

Give indications for Asafœtida in Iritis.

Syphilitic iritis, burning throbbing pains, soreness of bones around the eyes, relief from pressure on eye balls.

Give indications for Bryonia in Glaucoma.

Tension of eyeballs increased; hot tears flow from eye; photophobia and dimness of vision.

Give indications for Calcarea carb.?

Corneal opacities, scrofulous ophthalmia, pustules and ulcers on cornea, with general *Calcarea* symptoms.

Give symptoms calling for Kali hyd. in Syphilitic iritis?

After abuse of *Mercury*, when the symptoms are violent.

Give eye symptoms of Lachesis.

Dimness of vision, dim sight, evidence of heart disease and vertigo; retinal apoplexy.

FEVER (Simple).

Give in brief the indications for Aconite in Fevers.

Sthenic Fevers, with chilliness on the slightest movement; dry heat of skin, thirst, red cheeks, quickened respiration; full, bounding, rapid, tense pulse, with mental anxiety and aggravation towards evening. Every motion makes the patient chilly, but he is at the same time very restless from the mental anxiety.

When does Aconite cease to be of use?

In the second stage of inflammation; when it has localized itself.

How does Aconite differ from Veratrum viride in Fevers?

Veratrum viride has more arterial excitement and less nervous excitement than *Aconite*, and a characteristic of *Veratrum viride* is a bright red streak through the centre of the tongue.

When is Belladonna indicated in Fever?

When there are symptoms of delirium and cerebral excitement present, and a pungent heat of the skin.

The fevers of Gelsemium, what characterizes them?

Three D's: Drowsiness, Dullness and Dizziness; soreness of muscles and absence of thirst; great prostration and remission of symptoms.

What is the fever of Pulsatilla?

Chilliness predominates; fever without thirst, with oppression and sleepiness; worse about two or three in the afternoon.

Give four characteristics of Phosphorus in fever.

1. The adynamic, low type of fever.
2. The lack of thirst.
3. The periodicity—4 or 5 in the afternoon.
4. The sleepiness which accompanies.

How can Aconite, Apis and Gelsemium be differentiated in fevers in general?

Aconite typifies the synochal fever. *Gelsemium* typifies remittent or intermittent. *Apis* typifies intermittent or typhoid.

Mention some remedies having fever without thirst.

Apis, *Phos.*, *Puls.*, *China* and *Gelsem*.

What of the simple fever calling for Arsenicum?

It is fever belonging to intense local disease, to inflammation tending to destruction of tissue. There is anxiety, fear of death and restlessness.

When should Sulphur follow Aconite in fever?

When despite *Aconite* the dry heat continues; there is no perspiration; the patient becomes drowsy and restless, and tends to fall into a typhoid state from continuation of this heat.

Give fever of Bryonia.

Hard, tense pulse, intense headache, mouth dry, tongue coated white down middle; patient avoids light and motion. Thirst for large quantities of water at long intervals.

FISSURE OF ANUS.

What are the symptoms of Graphites in Fissure of the Anus?

Anus is extremely sore; stools covered with mucus; no tenesmus or constriction.

Give symptoms for Pæonia.

Fissures with a great deal of oozing; the anus is moist, sore and smarting all the time.

Give indications for Nitric acid.

Fissure with a sensation as if splinters or sticks were in the anus; much tenesmus and constriction.

When would Silicea be indicated :

When the characteristic irritability of the sphincter is present and the stool slips back when partially expelled.

Give indications for Ratanhia.

Where there is a great deal of constriction; anus aches and burns for hours after stool.

GANGRENE.

When is Arsenicum the remedy in Gangrene?

There is great relief from warmth. Dry gangrene of old people, with soreness and burning in the parts affected.

How does Arsenicum differ from Secale, another great Gangrene remedy?

Secale has relief from cold applications. It is useful in the same kind of dry gangrene of old people.

What is the remedy for Carbuncles and Boils which become gangrenous?

Carbo veg.

GASTRIC DERANGEMENTS.

What are the grand characteristics of Nux vomica in Dyspepsia?

When it is caused by mental overwork where there is distress in the stomach, coming on an hour or so after meals, and where the patient is cranky and irascible, and where he has a dull frontal headache in the morning. There is often nausea, empty retching and sour eructations.

What drugs have distress which commences immediately after eating?

Lycopodium, *Nux moschata* and *Abies nigra*.

What drugs besides Nux are often indicated in the flatulent Dyspepsia of drunkards and those who use alcoholic stimulants?

Carbo veg. and *Sulphur*.

What is the characteristic drug for Dyspepsia of beer drinkers?

Kali bichromicum.

What is an indicating symptom for Nux vom. in an attack of Dyspepsia?

Abnormal hunger, which precedes the attack for several days.

What drug has the symptom that vomiting occurs three or four hours after the patient eats?

Kreosote.

What drugs have pain and tenderness in the pit of the stomach, with aggravation at eleven o'clock in the morning?

Sepia, *Sulphur* and *Natrum carbonicum*..

What is the characteristic tongue of Nux in dyspeptic troubles?

It is usually coated white, especially on the posterior part.

What are the special desires and aversions of Nux?

There is a strong desire for beer and bitters and an aversion to coffee.

What are the characteristic symptoms of Carbo veg. in dyspepsia?

There is a slow and imperfect digestion. A weight in the stomach and a faint, gone feeling, which is not relieved by eating; after eating a few mouthfuls there is a sense of repletion. There is a great deal of burning in the stomach which extends to the back. There is a distention of the stomach and bowels, which is temporarily relieved by belching. There is heaviness, fullness and sleepiness after eating, and the flatulence causes asthmatic breathing and dyspnœa. The patient may even desire to be fanned.

What are some of the causes of Dyspepsia that would especially indicate Carbo vegetabilis?

Dyspepsias from overeating or high living; useful in the chronic dyspepsias of the aged; or in stomach troubles from abuse of *Alcohol*.

How does the flatulence of Carbo veg. differ from that of Lycopodium?

Carbo veg. flatulence is more of the stomach, while that of *Lyc.* is more of the intestines.

What other drugs have heaviness, fullness and sleepiness after eating?

Nux moschata and *Lycopodium*.

How does Carbo veg. differ in general from Sulphuric acid?

Carbo veg. is a putrid remedy, and indicated in putrid dyspepsia. *Sulphuric acid* is a sour remedy and indicated in acid conditions.

In the pressure caused by flatulence, how does Carbo veg. compare with China and Nux vom?

It has more upward pressure on the diaphragm, causing oppression of breathing, while *China* has not so much downward pressure as *Nux vom*.

Give another distinguishing feature between Carbo veg. and Lyc.

Under *Carbo veg.* there is a tendency to diarrhœa. Under *Lyc.* the tendency is to constipation.

What are the symptoms of China in dyspepsia?

There is distention of the stomach, momentarily relieved by belching. There are sour or bitter eructations. There is slow digestion, and the patient faints easily. There is a sensation as if the food had lodged in the œsophagus behind the sternum. The food seems to lie a long time in the stomach and causes eructations, and is finally vomited undigested. The distention after eating a little is characteristic.

What other drug has the sensation as if the food had lodged in the œsophagus behind the sternum?

Pulsatilla.

What drug has a sensation as if a hard boiled egg lay in the stomach?

Abies nigra.

How is China distinguished from Carbo veg.?

Although useful in cases where there is depression of the vital powers, it does not have the belching nor the burning which *Carbo veg.* has.

What are the symptoms of Lycopodium in Dyspepsia?

The patient has a vigorous appetite. After eating a small quantity of food, he feels so full and bloated that he has to force himself to take another mouthful. The distress is felt immediately upon eating. The patient is very sleepy after eating. There is a great deal of flatulence in the stomach and intestines, which presses upward and causes difficulty of breathing. Ravenous hunger, which if not satisfied causes headache, sour taste, sour belching and sometimes sour vomiting.

What drugs have a distress which comes on about two hours after eating?

Pulsatilla, Nux vom. and *Anacardium.*

Under what drugs is this sensation of satiety after eating food?

Arsenic, Carbo veg., China, Sepia and *Sulphur.*

Does belching of gas in Lyc. relieve?

It does not.

How does Lyc. differ from Nux vom.?

The distress immediately after eating belongs to *Lyc.*, while in *Nux vom.* the flatus presses downward rather than upward. *Nux vom.* has constipation from fitful intestinal action. *Lyc.* from contraction of the sphincter.

What is the difference between Sepia and Lycopodium?

Sepia has a sensation of emptiness in the epigastrium, while *Lyc.* has a sensation of fullness. Both have red sand in the urine. That of *Sepia*, however, is very offensive.

What symptom has Lyc. that is similar to one found under Argentum nitricum?

A great desire for sweets.

What drug desires especially oysters?

Lachesis.

What characteristics has Pulsatilla in Dyspepsia?

Dryness of the mouth and putrid taste, and a sensation as if the food had lodged under the sternum. There is a feeling of fullness and weight in the stomach, which comes on an hour or two after eating. There is a great deal of flatulence, which characterizingly moves about, causing painful sensation about the chest, which is relieved by eructation. It is especially useful for dyspepsia arising from fatty foods, pork or pastry, or from chilling the stomach with ice cream or ice water. The eructations taste of the food. Tongue thickly white coated.

What other drugs have Dyspepsia arising from rich and fatty food?

Ipecac., Thuja and *Carbo veg.*

What other drugs have stomach symptoms caused from chilling the stomach?

Arsenic and *Carbo veg.*

How is Pulsatilla distinguished from Nux vom?

Firstly, by the mental condition. Then *Pulsatilla* is worse in the evening and *Nux vom.* is worse in the morning. *Pulsatilla* has more heartburn and *Nux vom.* more water brash.

Give the stomach symptoms of Antimonium crudum.

Nausea and persistent vomiting occurring as soon as

the child eats or drinks. Digestive troubles from overloading the stomach; a useful remedy for the ill effects of Thanksgiving or Christmas dinners; there is the white tongue and the vomited matters containing food, and there is a great deal of fullness, distress and distention about the abdomen; eructations tasting of food.

Give the symptoms for Anacardium.

There is a sickening feeling, which comes on about two hours after eating, and a dull pain in the stomach, which extends to the spine. The great characteristic of the drug is a great relief of all the symptoms after eating. The patient is forced to eat to relieve these symptoms. Tasteless or sour eructations.

What other three drugs have relief from eating?

Petroleum, *Chelidonium* and *Graphites*.

Under what condition is Petroleum indicated?

There is ravenous hunger and gastralgia relieved by eating; it being especially useful in long, lingering gastric troubles with a great deal of nausea. Aversion to fat food and meat. Indigestion from *sauer kraut*. The nausea is worse from riding and motion.

How does Anacardium differ from Nux vom.?

Both have urging to stool, but unlike *Nux vom.* in going to stool the desire passes away and there is a characteristic symptom of a plug in the rectum.

What would indicate Chelidonium in Dyspepsia?

For this drug to be effective, liver symptoms must be prominent.

What drug has Gastralgia which is worse from eating?

Argentum nitricum.

What are the symptoms of Sepia in Dyspepsia?

There is a feeling of goneness in the stomach; not relieved by eating. There is a white coated tongue and sour or putrid taste in the mouth. There is nausea at the sight or smell of food. The *Sepia* patient is worse in the morning and evening. There is a great longing for acids and pickles, and it is a useful remedy for dyspepsia from the overuse of tonics. Sensation of a lump in the stomach.

Give another drug having a sensation of goneness in the pit of the stomach which is not relieved by eating.

Carbo animalis.

What drug has nausea at the thought of food; even mention food and he vomits?

Colchicum.

What are some symptoms of Sulphur in Dyspepsia?

There is a bitter, sour taste and putrid eructation and sour vomiting. It is useful in flatulent dyspepsia, and it has a feeling of satiety after eating a small quantity of food, and it has an empty, gone feeling in the epigastrium about eleven o'clock. There is a great desire for sweets, which make him sick, causing a sour stomach and heartburn. There is canine hunger. The patient can hardly wait for meals and is forced to get up at night to eat.

What other drug has canine hunger, causing patient to get up at night and eat?

Phosphorus.

What drugs have a hungry, gnawing feeling in the epigastrium at about eleven o'clock in the morning?

Natrum carb. and *Natrum sulph.*

What are the characteristic symptoms of Phosphorus in the stomach troubles?

A craving for cold food and drink, which relieves momentarily, but which are vomited as soon as they become warm in the stomach; there are sour eructations and a white tongue. In chronic dyspepsia where the patient vomits as soon as food strikes the stomach it is the remedy. Perforating ulcer of stomach vomiting of coffee-ground-like matters.

What other drug has this symptom of vomiting as soon as food reaches the stomach?

Bismuth.

Give symptoms of Natrum carb. in Dyspepsia.

There is hypochondriasis, morning nausea and empty retchings; sour eructations and fetid flatulence and a weak, hungry feeling in the epigastrium at eleven o'clock A. M. The patient is low-spirited after a meal and is worse after vegetable or starchy food, and it is especially useful in dyspepsia from eating soda discuits.

How does Natrum carb. stand in relation to Nux vom. and Sepia?

It stands between them.

What are the symptoms of Kali carb. in Dyspepsia?

Dyspepsia of weak, anæmic and easily exhausted patients who have a tired feeling and backache. There is a faint, sickening feeling in the epigastrium before eating, sour eructations, heartburn and a weak, nervous sensation. The patient is sleepy while eating, and after eating there is an undue flatulence; everything he eats seems to turn to gas. All the symptoms of *Kali carb.* are aggravated by soup or by coffee.

What other remedies have the symptoms that everything eaten turns to gas?

Argentum nitricum and *Iodine*.

What drugs also have Dyspepsia from loss of fluids, or from protracted illness?

China and *Carbo veg.*

What are the indications for Graphites in Dyspepsia?

Tympanitic distention of the stomach; the patient is obliged to loosen his clothing; burning pains and cramps and putrid eructations; there is a burning, crampy pain, which is relieved by eating; there is disagreeable taste in the morning, and aversion to meat.

Compare Lycopodium here.

Lycopodium has distention with great accumulation of flatus; but this flatus is not rancid or putrid as under *Graphites*.

What drugs have the symptom that the patient has to loosen the clothing after eating?

Lycopodium, *Carbo veg.*, *Nux vom.* and *China*.

What drugs have aversion to meat?

All chlorotic remedies, such as *Ferrum* and *China*.

What drug has an intense desire for coffee?

Angustura.

Give the stomach symptoms of Ipecac.

Intense nausea and vomiting, which is followed by exhaustion and sleepiness. Troubles arising from fat food, pork, pastry, candy, etc. The stomach has a hanging down, relaxed feeling.

What distinguishes it from Antimonium crud. in stomach troubles?

The tongue is clean, whereas in *Antimonium crud.* it is thickly coated white.

What other drugs have a relaxed hanging down feeling at the stomach?

Staphisagria, *Tabacum* and *Sepia*.

How is Pulsatilla distinguished in gastric troubles?

The distress in *Pulsatilla* comes on while the food is still in the stomach; with *Ipecac* it is while the stomach is empty; the tongue, too, with *Ipecac* is clean, in *Pulsatilla* coated.

What are the stomach symptoms of Hydrastis?

There is a sinking, gone feeling at the pit of the stomach; an empty, gone feeling, as if the patient had suffered from a diarrhœa for a long time; there are also eructations and some nausea. Atonic dyspepsia; tongue large, flabby, slimy.

Give the indications for Argentum nitricum in gastric troubles.

The patient craves candies or sweets, which disagree; there is flatulence, which presses up and causes dyspnœa; there are violent efforts to belch, and the gas rises to a certain point, when a sudden spasmodic contraction prevents its escaping, but it is finally expelled in loud reports. There is severe gastralgia, the pains radiate from the stomach in all directions; they are relieved by hard pressure and by bending double; the pains often increase gradually, and decrease gradually as under *Stannum;* vomiting of glairy mucus relieves.

How does Bismuth compare in this Gastralgia?

In *Bismuth* it is purely nervous gastralgia, and as soon as the least food touches the stomach the patient vomits. Cold drinks relieve.

What are the stomach symptoms of Staphisagria?

A sensation as if the stomach was hanging down, relaxed; it seems to be flabby and weak; a great desire for wine, brandy or tobacco. Pain in abdomen after every morsel of food or drink.

What other drug has similar symptoms?

Ipecac.

What is the chief characteristic symptom of Robinia?

Acid dyspepsia with weight in the stomach and eructations of a sour fluid; intensely acid vomiting, it sets the teeth on edge.

What are the stomach characteristics of Sulphuric acid?

Extreme sourness of all vomited matters; the stomach feels cold and relaxed, and the patient desires a stimulating drink, such as brandy; the stomach is so weak that all food is vomited. Stomach troubles of inebriates with these symptoms are greatly benefited by the remedy.

What are the stomach symptoms of Arsenicum?

Burning, griping pains in the stomach followed by

great prostration and vomiting; the vomiting is severe; the patient vomits water as soon as it becomes warm in the stomach; the stomach is very irritable, and it is a remedy for irritable stomachs of drunkards; there is heartburn and gulping up of a watery substance.

What are the digestive symptoms of Bryonia?

Food distresses the patient as soon as he takes it; it lies in the stomach like a hard load; there is a white or yellowish-white coating on the tongue; there is a faint, weak feeling on sitting up.

What is the sphere of action of Cadmium sulphate?

It is a cross between *Arsenic* and *Bryonia*, and comes in between those two drugs in certain stomach conditions where we have the characteristic *Arsenic* symptoms, and a desire to keep perfectly quiet, as under *Bryonia*.

Give the stomach symptoms of Calcarea.

Pressure in the stomach, the pit is swollen like a saucer turned bottom side up; sour vomiting and ravenous hunger in the morning; the patient cannot bear anything tight about the waist.

What are the stomach symptoms of Hepar?

Craving for acids, alcoholics and strong tasting substances; hunger and gnawing in the stomach; cannot bear anything tight about the waist.

What are the indications for the use of Abies Canadensis?

There is a gnawing or burning in the stomach, a hungry, faint, weak feeling with craving for indigestible or unsuitable articles of food

What is the great characteristic of Abies nigra?

A sensation as if the patient had swallowed some indigestible substance which had stuck in the cardiac extremity of the stomach; a hard boiled egg sensation; dyspepsia from abuse of tobacco.

Give the stomach symptoms and cravings of Alumina.

Constriction on swallowing food, and the patient is always worse after eating potatoes; there is craving for chalk, charcoal, slate pencils and other indigestible substances.

What are the dyspeptic symptoms of Arnica?

Throbbing headache and drowsiness after a meal; tendency to putrescence, foul breath, shiny tongue, belching of gas which tastes like rotten eggs; tympanitic distention of the abdomen, foul-smelling stool and a great deal of weakness.

What are the stomach symptoms of Ferrum met.?

There seems to be no secretion in the stomach capable of changing the food, and it is vomited as taken. The appetite is ravenous.

What are the digestive and bilious symptoms of Iris versicolor?

Severe burning distress in the stomach, vomiting of food, vomiting of excessively acid substances, with distress over the liver.

What are the digestive symptoms of Ignatia?

Bitter taste in the mouth and regurgitation of a bitter fluid, gastralgia and hiccough, relieved by eating and smoking. Empty, gone feeling and great nervous depression; empty retching, relieved by eating; the patient vomits simple food, but retains such things as cabbage.

Give the stomach symptoms of Kali muriaticum.

Dyspepsia, with white tongue; pain after eating; liver sluggish; fatty food disagrees; indigestion, with vomiting of a whitish mucus, with gathering of water in the mouth.

What are the gastric symptoms of Kali bichromicum?

Bitter vomiting, mixed with mucus, renewed by every attempt to eat or drink; fullness even after eating a small quantity, worse from meat; dyspepsia from beer.

Give the gastric symptoms of Calcarea phosphorica.

Excessive flatulence; the patient craves ham, bacon, salted or smoked meats. Enlarged mesenteric glands; pain after a small quantity of food.

What are the digestive characteristics of Colchicum?

Extreme aversion to food, nausea and loathing at the thought of food; he gags at the mere mention of food; loss of appetite, great debility and brown tongue.

What are the digestive symptoms of Cyclamen?

Aggravation from fat food, desire for lemonade, and thirst; otherwise similar to *Pulsatilla*.

What are the stomach symptoms of Belladonna?

Pain in the stomach, worse during a meal. Gastralgia, pains go to spine, not much thirst.

What are the stomach symptoms of Natrum muriaticum?

There is a violent thirst; aversion to bread; water brash and feeling of weakness and sinking in the stomach.

What are the stomach symptoms of Asafœtida?

Belching of rancid gas, and an empty, gone feeling in the stomach in the forenoon; greasy taste; burning in the stomach and œsophagus; great meteorismus.

Give the stomach symptoms of Natrum phos. and indications as given by Schuessler.

Great acidity, sour risings, vomiting of sour fluids with pain in the stomach and great flatulence. The sourness is the characteristic of the drug.

What is the indication of the tongue?

It has a thick, yellow coating on the back part.

Give an indication for Salicylic acid.

Dyspepsia, with excessive accumulation of flatulence and acidity of the stomach; much belching of gas.

Give an indication for Carbolic acid.

Flatulence of the aged depending upon imperfect digestion; acidity and burning in the stomach.

GLANDULAR TROUBLES.

What are the symptoms of Carbo animalis in the glandular system?

Induration of the glands, inguinal and axillary, particularly of syphilitic origin; when the induration is hard as a stone, and when the tissues surrounding them are also hard.

What are some indications for Iodine in glandular troubles?

In goitre, an enlargement of the thyroid gland, it is a

What are the general glandular symptoms of Silicea?

useful remedy; also in orchitis, with pains extending to the abdomen.

What are the general glandular symptoms of Silicea?

It is the remedy in suppurating glandular affections, such as inflammation of the breasts and in inflammation and suppuration of the inguinal glands or suppurative conditions about the salivary glands.

What form of glandular disease calls for Conium?

Adenometa, glands of stony hardness, with little or no pain; beginning of scirrhus.

Give glandular symptoms of Bromine.

Glands enlarged, indurated, tend to suppurate with excoriating discharge and persistent hardness of gland around opening; undue heat and warmth in glands.

Mention some remedies useful for induration of axillary glands.

Belladonna (especially at climaxis), *Carbo an.*, *Bromine* and *Calc. carb.*

Mention some remedies for indurated Buboes.

Alumina, *Badiaga* and *Carbo an.*

What are the indications for Spongia?

Goitre, with suffocating spells at night; swelling and induration of the lymphatic glands.

GLEET.

When should Sulphur be given in Gleet?

In persons subject to catarrhs, where the case has been

maltreated by injections, and where there is much irritation and soreness and the urine burns the parts.

Give indications for Sepia.

Gleet with scanty discharge in the morning only.

When is Pulsatilla indicated in Gleet?

When the discharge is thick, yellow and bland; phlegmatic and scrofulous constitutions.

GONORRHŒA.

What are the male sexual symptoms of Argentum nitricum?

Gonorrhœa, thick, yellow, purulent discharge, with soreness of urethra; indifference during coitus, but sexual dreams with emissions.

What are the principal characteristics of Cannabis sativa?

Urethritis, with purulent discharge, great burning and tenderness on urinating; glans penis dark red and swollen; there may be chordee; there is also a spasmodic contraction of sphincter vesicæ on urinating.

When should Cantharis be preferred?

Where there is intense sexual excitement. Gonorrhœa, with intense irritation and persistent erections; the discharge is purulent and bloody; useful when the disease has been sent to the bladder by injections.

Give a distinguishing feature between these two remedies.

Cantharis has more tenesmus. *Cannabis sat.* has more burning and smarting.

Give symptoms indicating Copaiva in Urethritis.

Burning in the neck of bladder and urethra; catarrh of

bladder with great dysuria following gonorrhœa; there is swelling of the orifice of the urethra and constant desire to urinate; urine smells of violets, especially in gonorrhœa; discharge yellow, purulent and corrosive; hæmaturia.

How does Cubeba compare here?

Cubeba has cutting and constriction after micturition; urinates every ten or fifteen minutes, with smarting tenesmus and ropy mucus; useful in inflamed prostate.

When is Mercury indicated in Gonorrhœa?

Green, purulent discharge; worse at night; with swollen prepuce, phymosis or paraphymosis.

What are the indications for Mercurius corrosivus in Gonorrhœa?

Green, purulent discharge, worse at night; the meatus is dark red and there is violent tenesmus of the bladder.

What are the sexual symptoms of Natrum sulphuricum?

It is one of the principal remedies in sycosis, especially where there are condylomata.

What are the symptoms of Thuja in Gonorrhœa?

Thin, greenish discharge, scalding urination, warts and condylomata about the genitals, gonorrhœa suppressed by injections, and complicated with rheumatism or orchitis.

Give indications for Digitalis.

Burning in urethra with purulent discharge, bright yellow in color. Glans penis is inflamed, with a copious secretion of thick pus over its surface.

When is Gelsemium indicated?

In the beginning, where there is great urethral soreness; burning along urethra.

What remedy is useful for a sudden irresistible desire to urinate?

Petroselinum.

When is Pulsatilla indicated?

Discharge is thick, muco-purulent, yellowish or yellowish green. Pains in the groins, going across hypogastrium from side to side. Suppression of discharge with resulting orchitis.

Give indications for Sulphur.

Burning and smarting during urination; bright redness of the lips of the meatus urinarius. Phymosis with induration of prepuce.

GOUT.

When is Colchicum indicated in Gout?

Where the swelling is red or pale, with extreme tenderness to touch and a tendency to shift about from joint to joint; pains are worse in the evening and from the slightest motion; metastasis of gout to heart, with cutting pains about heart and oppression.

Give indications for Ammonium phosphoricum in Gout.

Constitutional gout with nodes and concretions in the joints; chronic cases where these concretions of Urate of Soda deform the joints.

What are the symptoms calling for Arnica in Gout?

Extreme soreness.

What of the use of Ledum?

Pains worse from the warmth of the bed; drawing pains in joints; scanty effusion, which tends to harden into nodosities.

How does Bryonia compare?

Ledum produces a scanty effusion, which tends to harden into nodosities, while *Bryonia* tends to a copious effusion.

Give some other remedies having nodular swellings in the joints.

Calcarea carb., *Benzoic acid*, *Lycopodium*, *Lithium carb.* and *Antimonium crud.*

Give symptoms of Guaiacum in Gout.

Concretions of the joints. Gouty inflammation of the knee with abscess. Contractions of muscles.

HAY FEVER.

Give indications for Arsenicum in Hay Fever.

Continual sneezing, which gives no relief. Discharge thin and acrid. The patient cannot lie down, especially after midnight. There is dyspnœa.

How does Sinapis nigra compare?

The mucous membrane of the nose is dry and hot; there is no discharge.

Give symptoms calling for Ranunculus bulbosus.

Smarting in eyes; nose stuffed up towards evening with

pressure at the root and tingling and crawling in nasal cavity; also hoarseness.

When is Sabadilla the remedy?

When there are violent paroxysms of sneezing, with great irritation and itching of the Schneiderian membrane.

HEMORRHAGES.

What are the hemorrhagic symptoms of Phosphorus?

The hemorrhagic diathesis; the blood does not coagulate; hemoptysis and hematemesis.

When is Secale useful in uterine Hemorrhage?

Passive, painless flow of dark liquid blood, the patient is wrinkled and scrawny, is often unconscious and cold, hemorrhages preceded by formication and tingling. Slightest motion aggravates flow.

When is Cinchona indicated in Hemorrhages?

Dark clotted hemorrhages, from any part of the body, with coldness of face, collapse, gasping for breath, and the patient wants to be fanned; ringing in the ears.

What other drug has a copious passive Hemorrhage and where the patient desires to be fanned?

Carbo veg.

Give the unique symptoms of Acalypha Indica.

Dry cough, followed by spitting of blood, which is pure in the morning, but dark, lumpy and clotted in the evening, with a constricted feeling around the chest.

What are the main characteristic symptoms of Sabina?

Metrorrhagia, with paroxysmal flow of bright color, accompanied by pains in the joints. After abortion or labor, pains in back to pubis.

What are the Hemorrhages of Ipecac?

In hæmoptysis, where the blood is bright and in gushes, with nausea and gagging. In hemorrhages of bright red blood, which flows steadily; nausea, etc.

What are the symptoms indicating Lachesis in Hemorrhages?

Hemorrhages of dark blood, which deposits a sediment as of charred straw; small wounds bleed profusely and the blood remains fluid, does not coagulate.

What is the Hemorrhage of Belladonna?

It is bright red from the uterus and characteristically *hot*.

What are the indications for Bovista in Hemorrhages?

Hemorrhages from relaxation of the capillary system; epistaxis or menstrual hemorrhages, where the blood flows with very little exertion; the flow occurs more at night or in the morning.

What are the symptoms calling for Ustilago in Hemorhages?

Bright, partly clotted hemorrhages from passive congestion of the uterus; hemorrhages from slight causes, as from digital examinations.

What is our principal use of Millefolium?

In hemorrhages from any part of the body of bright red

blood, and occurring after mechanical injuries. Hæmoptysis, epistaxis or hemorrhages from the uterus or bowels.

How does it differ from Aconite here?

Aconite has anxiety; *Millefolium* not.

What are the characterizing features of Erigeron, another member of the same family, in Hemorrhages?

The hemorrhage is of bright red blood and is increased by every motion of the patient.

Give Hemorrhage calling for Cinnamomum.

Profuse hemorrhage from a strain or misstep; tendency to hemorrhages; frequent attacks of nosebleed.

What is the Hemorrhage of Trillium pendulum?

Active or passive; threatened abortion, with a gush of blood on each movement, with a sensation as if the hips and back were falling apart; relieved by bandaging the hips tightly.

Give indications for Carbo veg. in Nosebleed.

Persistent, dark, occurring in old and debilitated persons, the face being pale, sunken, almost hippocratic; nosebleed in old people.

What remedy has Nosebleed where the blood coagulates and hangs from the nose like icicles?

Mercurius.

When is Ferrum indicated?

It stands between *China* and *Ipecac*. It suits anæmic cases like *China*, where there is much prostration, and it has bright red, gushing flow and difficulty of breathing, like *Ipecac*.

Give hemorrhagic symptoms of Hamamelis.

The flow is dark, passive, venous and accompanied by a feeling of soreness, and the patient is greatly exhausted.

What of Phosphorus in Hemorrhages?

Hemorrhagic diathesis. Hemorrhages from any part of body, especially from lungs or stomach.

Mention a few drugs for Hæmoptysis with brief indications.

Aconite: Bright red, with great anxiety and fever.
Cactus: With strong throbbing of heart, less fever and anxiety than *Aconite*.
Millefolium: Bright red, no fever.

Mention two drugs having Hemorrhage due to tissue degeneration.

Arsenic and *Carbo veg*.

What are the Hemorrhages of Crocus?

Epistaxis or other hemorrhage where the blood is thick and dark, hangs in strings from nose.

HEMORRHOIDS.

What are the indications for Aloes in Hemorrhoids?

They protrude like a bunch of grapes after each stool, and are relieved by the application of cold water and aggravated by motion.

How does Aloes compare with Collinsonia in Hemorrhoids?

Collinsonia most always has constipation and *Aloes* diarrhœa.

What is our principal use of Æsculus?

Abdominal plethora, throbbing deep in the abdomen. Hemorrhoids accompanied by a feeling of dryness in the rectum as though little sticks, splinters or burrs were sticking in the mucous membrane. They are purple in color and accompanied by backache. Feeling of fulness in the rectum as if it would protrude. Bowels loose.

What drug has a symptom that the Rectum seems as if full of pounded glass?

Ratanhia; another symptom of this drug is that the anus aches and burns for hours after stool.

What are the Hemorrhoids of Collinsonia?

Where there is a sensation of sticks in the rectum; constipation, with prolapsus uteri and hemorrhoids.

What are the Hemorrhoidal symptoms of Nux?

Itching hemorrhoids, which keep the patient awake; bleeding piles, with ineffectual urging to stool.

Give Hemorrhoidal symptoms of Hamamelis.

Soreness is the great keynote. There is also much backache and hemorrhage.

What are the indications for Sulphur?

When the hemorrhoidal flow becomes suppressed and reflex troubles arise.

HEADACHE.

Give the symptoms of Belladonna in Headache.

The pain is worse on right side and worse in the frontal region, aggravated by lying down. There is a great deal of throbbing, the pain sometimes being of a stabbing, sharp character, driving the patient almost wild; greatly aggravated by light, noise or jarring. There is apt to be a red face accompanying the headache.

Give three differentiating symptoms between Sanguinaria and Belladonna in Headache.

Belladonna has hot head, more throbbing, flushed face, and cold feet.

Belladonna is relieved by being propped up in bed, while *Sanguinaria* has relief from lying down.

Belladonna has not so marked, the pain coming up over the head from the occiput, and *Sanguinaria* is more useful in the gastric form.

Give the symptoms of Sanguinaria in Headache.

Genuine sick headache; pain beginning in morning and in the occiput, crosses up over the head and settles in the right eye. The patient can neither tolerate noise nor light and only sleep relieves. When the pain is at its acme there is vomiting. The vomited matters consist of food and bile. Temporal veins distended.

What is the Headache of Iris versicolor?

Periodical headaches with intense throbbing, supraorbital pains, and accompanying the headache there is temporary blindness. At the height of the headache vomiting occurs, vomited matters being bitter or sour, or both. It is especially a remedy for headaches of school teachers, college professors and students. Hemicrania commencing with blurring of vision.

What is the Headache of Spigelia?

Spigelia holds the same relation to the left side of the head that *Silicea* does to the right side. The pains settle over the left eye and are neuralgic in character. The pains are apt to follow the course of the sun, beginning in the morning, reaching the acme at noon, and generally subsiding at sunset. There is a sensation as if the head were open along the vertex. Worse from noise, jar or thinking.

What drug has a pain in the back of the head as if it were alternately opening and closing?

Cocculus

What are some other symptoms of Cocculus in Headache?

The headache is in the occipital region in lower part of the back of the head and in the nape of the neck. It is one of our principal headache remedies when in the occipital region. Vertigo is a marked symptom.

Mention some other remedies useful for occipital Headaches.

Gelsemium, *Juglans cathartica*, *Bryonia*, *Petroleum*, *Carbo veg.* and *Nux vomica*.

What is the Headache of Silicea?

The *Silicea* headache is a nervous headache, and it is caused by excessive mental exertion. It is supra-orbital and worse over right eye. Worse from noise, motion or jars, and better from wrapping the head up warmly.

The pains come up from back of the neck into the head.

How does the Headache of Menyanthes compare here?

It commences at nape and comes up over head, there is a bursting pain as if the skull would burst open. Pressure, rather than warmth, relieves; worse by going up stairs, when there is a sensation of weight on vertex.

What is the difference between the Headache of Silicea and the Headache of Argentum nitricum?

The headache of *Argentum nitricum* is better from wrapping the head up, not so much from the heat as from the pressure. The difference is that while heat relieves *Silicea* headache, pressure relieves *Argentum nitricum* headache.

Mention some other symptoms of Argentum nitricum in Headache.

There is a sensation as if the head were enormously large, and it is accompanied with much vertigo. The pains increase to such a degree that the patient almost loses her senses.

Give the Headache of Melilotus alba.

It is a headache which almost drives the patient frantic. There are intense throbbing pains through the head. It seems as if the brain would burst through the forehead. It is especially useful in congestive variety of headaches.

What is the Headache of Cinchona?

Headache with violent throbbing of the carotids; head feels as though skull would burst; sensation as if brain beat in waves against skull; anæmic headache.

How does this compare with the Belladonna Headache?

The headache and throbbing of carotids so characteristic of *Belladonna* is due to hyperæmia, while under *Cinchona* it is an anæmic condition.

What drug has the sensation as if the vertex were pressed asunder and the patient must hold it together?

Carbo animalis.

What is the Headache of Paris quadrifolia?

A headache of spinal origin and a sensation as if the head were immensely large.

What is the Headache of Theridion?

A sick headache, especially in hysterical women where the great key-note is sensitiveness to noise, nausea and aggravation from motion. The headache is apt to be periodical and over the left eye, throbbing and shooting.

What is the Headache of Nux vomica?

It is a headache due to gastric troubles, and it occurs in the morning. The headache is either in the occiput or over one or the other eye, and is often associated with vomiting of food and violent retching; also a bilious occipital headache. Headaches of high livers; in those who use alcohol to excess, often associated with constipation and hemorrhoids.

What drug has a Headache as from beating of little hammers in the head and worse from moving the head or eyeballs?

Natrum muriaticum.

What is the Headache of Sepia?

It is a sharp pain in the lower part of the brain which shoots upward. The patient can bear neither light nor noise. It is usually accompanied with uterine discharges and often by nausea and vomiting. Headaches relieved by sleep or violent motion.

Give Headache of Carbolic acid.

A feeling of fulness, mostly in the frontal region, and especially supra-orbital. Sometimes with pain in the eyeballs. This fulness may become excessive, progress to unconsciousness even uræmic or apoplectiform in character.

What is the Headache of Gelsemium?

Dull, heavy ache with heavy eyelids. It commences in the nape, passes over the head and settles in an eye; worse in the morning, relieved by a discharge of urine; the patient is listless and stupid, the face is dark red, appears as if under the influence of liquor; there is also a feeling of a band around the head.

Mention some other drugs having this last symptom.

Iodine, Mercury, Carbolic acid and *Sulphur*.

What other drugs have Headaches relieved by copious urination?

Aconite, Silicea, Veratrum album and *Ignatia*.

What drugs have Headaches with partial blindness?

Gelsemium, Natrum mur., Iris versicolor, Causticum, Psorinum and *Silicea*.

What are the head symptoms of Ignatia?

Heaviness in the head as if congested, relieved by stooping; there is a pain as if a nail were driven into the parietal or occipital region; clavus hystericus; the headache ends in vomiting or in a copious discharge of pale urine. It is aggravated by smoking or smelling tobacco.

What drugs have a sensation as if a nail were being driven into the occiput?

Thuja and *Coffea*.

What drug has a Headache as though a nail were being driven into the vertex or one or the other frontal eminence?

Thuja.

Give Headache of Bryonia.

The pain begins in the occiput or else in the forehead and goes back to the occiput. It is worse in morning and is aggravated by any motion. Each movement or motion of the eyeballs aggravates the pain. Splitting frontal headache extending backward and down neck, shoulders and back.

What other drug has a Headache with soreness of the eyeballs when moving?

Gelsemium.

How do Spigelia, Silicea and Carbo veg. compare with Bryonia?

Spigelia. Pain darting from behind, from and through left eyeball.

Silicea. Pain coming up from the nape of the neck through the occiput and over the vertex, and so down upon the forehead.

Carbo veg. Dull heavy pain extending through the base of the brain from the occiput to the supra-orbital region.

What is the Headache of Ipecac?

It is a headache of rheumatic origin, with a sensation as if the bones of the head were crushed or bruised. This crushed or bruised sensation extends to the root of the tongue and is accompanied with deathly nausea and vomiting.

What is the Headache of Cimicifuga?

There is a sensation as if the top of the head would fly off. There are sharp, lancinating pains in and over the eyes, shooting up to the top of the head. Under this remedy we have also a sensation as if the brain were moving in waves and a sharp pain extending from the occiput to the frontal region, as if a bolt were being driven through the head.

What is the Headache of Glonoine?

Throbbing headache, which may be in any part of the head. It seems as if the blood-vessels would burst, and every throb of the heart increases the pain.

Give the general differences between Glonoine and Belladonna.

The differences are these: *Glonoine* is relieved from uncovering; the headache is worse from bending the head backward; is relieved in the open air; cannot keep still; must walk about; no flushing of the face. *Belladonna* is worse from uncovering; better from bending the head backwards; worse in the open air, and better by holding the head still; face flushed.

What is the characteristic Headache of Palladium?

It is a headache which extends across the top of the head from ear to ear, accompanied by mental fatigue and a great deal of irritability.

What is the Headache of Phellandrium?

A pain as though a weight were on top of the head, and it involves the nerves going to the eyes; there is burning of the eyes and lachrymation.

What is the characteristic Headache of Rhus tox.?

It is a headache as if a board were strapped on to the frontal region; aching in occipital protuberances with much soreness of scalp.

What is the Headache of Kali bichromicum?

Periodical supra-orbital headache; as the headache starts the sight becomes lost, but it returns as the headache increases; it is more on the right side.

What are the head symptoms of Hepar?

Headache as if a nail were being driven into the right side of the head; offensive eruptions on the scalp. with non-excoriating discharges and great tenderness.

What other drugs have Headache as if a nail were being driven into the head?

Ignatia, as if driven into the top of the head; *Thuja*, as if driven into the frontal eminence.

What is the Headache of Selenium?

A nervous headache over the left eye, worse from the heat of the sun, and especially is it useful in headaches due to excessive use of *tea*.

When is Natrum carb. indicated in Headache?

When caused by walking in the sun. Dullness of the head. Patient is greatly fatigued by a short walk.

What is the peculiar head symptom of Cannabis Indica?

There is a sensation as if the head were opening and shutting along the vertex.

What are the head symptoms of Lachesis?

Headache over the left eye accompanying a cold, but as soon as discharge is established headache is better.

What are the head symptoms of Coffea?

Congestions, with excited state of the mind; headache, as if a nail had been driven into the parietal bone; worse in open air; hemicrania.

What is the characteristic head symptoms of Antimonium crudum?

Headache from bathing; all symptoms of the drug are worse from bathing. Headache from deranged stomach.

Give Headache of Onosmodium?

Pain in occiput with vertigo. Headaches caused by straining the eyes, with strained feeling in the eyes.

What are the special characteristic head symptoms or head indications of Natrum sulphuricum?

It is a useful remedy for ill effects of falls and injuries to the head, and especially so if mental troubles arise therefrom.

What are the head symptoms of Apis?

In meningitis it is indicated by the shrill outcries in sleep, and especially if due to a suppressed eruption.

What peculiar symptom has Oleander in the head?

Headache relieved by looking sideways.

What is the Headache of Aloes?

Dull headache across the forehead or a weight on the vertex; heaviness in the eyelids and nausea, relief from partially closing the eyes.

What is the characteristic Headache of Ferrum?

It is a throbbing headache at the base of the brain. It seems as if the head would burst; there is congestion and pulsating in the head, worse after midnight, with red face and cold feet.

What is the Headache of Anacardium?

Tearing headache from mental exertion; pains in forehead and back part of head, or a sensation as if a plug were in some part of the head. There is much mental irritability with these headaches.

When is Phosphoric acid indicated?

In headaches of school-girls, coming on and continuing as long as they study.

What are the Headaches of Pulsatilla?

Either gastric, rheumatic or uterine; mostly frontal or supra-orbital; worse by warmth and mental exertion, and worse in the evening. May be wandering pains, from one part of the head to another.

HEART, AFFECTIONS OF.

What are the symptoms of Aconite in heart diseases?

There is palpitation and anxiety with intense pain in the region of the heart, shooting down the left arm accompanied by a numbness and tingling in the fingers. It is the principal remedy in uncomplicated hypertrophy of the heart.

What other drugs have numbness of the left arm and shoulder in heart troubles?

Kalmia, Rhus tox. and *Pulsatilla.*

What drug has sensation as though the left arm were tightly bandaged to the body?

Actea racemosa.

What drug has the same symptom in the right arm that Aconite, Kalmia and Rhus tox. have in the left arm?

Phytolacca.

What are the indications for Rhus tox. in heart troubles?

There is palpitation of the heart when especially caused by over-exertion, and a weak feeling in the chest. It is a remedy for hypertrophy of the heart, especially if there be a rheumatic diathesis.

Give the heart symptoms of Kalmia.

The pains in the heart are sharp, taking away the breath, almost suffocating the patient. They shoot down into the abdomen or stomach. The pulse is very slow; not quite as slow as the pulse of *Digitalis*, however. It is the remedy for heart affections following gout or rheumatism. Numbness and tingling of left arm.

Give the heart symptoms of Digitalis.

The pulse is slow, but primarily strong. There is great weakness of the cardiac tissues, and secondarily the pulse becomes weak. Extra exertion increases its rapidity, but its force is diminished. The quick pulse becomes irregular and even intermittent. The heart feels as if the blood stood still. There is weakness and numbness in the left arm. There is often blueness on the surface of the body and the patient fears that the heart will cease beating if he should make any motion.

How does Gelsemium compare in this last symptom?

Under *Gelsemium* the patient is suddenly aroused from

sleep with a feeling that the heart will stop beating, and feels as though he must move about in order to keep the heart in action. There is faintness when rising from a sitting posture.

What are the heart symptoms of Spongia?

The patient is aroused frequently from sleep as if smothering. There is a blowing sound over one or the other valve of the heart, and on pressing the hand on the chest there is communicated to it a purring feeling.

What are the heart symptoms of Spigelia?

There are sharp pains shooting from the heart to the back and radiating from the heart down the arm, over the chest and down the spine. There is palpitation, worse from any movement of the arm or body. There is a purring sensation felt over the cardiac region. These symptoms may be associated with neuralgia, especially of the left side of the head. The pulse is intermittent. The slightest motion of the arms or hands makes the patient worse. The pulse is not synchronous with the heart.

Give the heart symptoms of Arsenic.

Arsenic has a hypertrophy of the heart resulting from climbing high places, mountains, etc. The heart beat is too strong. It is audible to the patient himself. Worse at night. The pulse may be accelerated and weak. There may be palpitation with great irregularity of action.

What are the heart symptoms of Apis?

It is useful in cardiac inflammations and dropsy. There is dyspnœa and lancinating pains in the region of the heart.

What are the heart symptoms of Veratrum vir.?

It is simply a condition of intense arterial excitement, and is indicated by the rapid, full pulse.

Give the heart symptoms of Cactus?

There is a sensation in the heart as if it were grasped by an iron hand and squeezed; constricted sensation about the heart. It is a remedy for carditis and pericarditis. There is a feeling about the lower part of the chest as if bound by a cord.

What are the uses of Phosphorus in heart troubles?

It is useful for fatty degeneration of the heart. There is venous stagnation, puffiness of the face, especially under the eyelids. Heart troubles accompanying pneumonia also indicate this drug.

What other drug has hypertrophy of the heart and dilation of the right side of the heart?

Pulsatilla.

What are the indications for Conium in heart troubles?

Weakness here causes the pulse to be one moment full and regular and the next to be soft and irregular. There are sudden jerks or shocks about the heart.

What other drugs have sudden jerks or shocks about the heart?

Zincum and *Aurum.*

What drug has the symptom that the patient wakes up suddenly out of sleep with a sensation as if respiration had ceased?

Grindelia.

What is the action of Kali hydriodicum?

It produces a smothering feeling about the heart, wakening the patient from sleep and compelling him to get out of bed.

What other drugs have this symptom?

Lachesis, Kali bich., Lactuca, Euphrasia and *Graphites.*

What are the heart symptoms of Lachesis?

There is oppression of the chest, inability to lie down and smothering feeling on awakening from sleep.

What are the symptoms indicating Iodine in heart disease?

There is enlargement of the heart, palpitation and a feeling as if it were being squeezed by a firm hand.

What are the heart symptoms of Kali carb?

There is an irregular or intermittent pulse, or a very rapid and a very weak pulse. There are sharp stitching pains in the cardiac region, it is indicated late in cardiac diseases when there is a deposit in the valves.

What are the heart symptoms of Sulphur?

There seems to be too much blood in the heart and there is violent palpitation. The blood rushes into the heart and the contraction of the heart is not rapid enough to remove it. There is a shortness of breath and a sensation as if the heart were too large for the thoracic cavity.

What are the heart symptoms of Tabacum?

There is palpitation, paroxysms of suffocation and tightness across the upper part of the chest. The pulse is feeble and irregular. There is a sensation of trembling in the cardiac region and fluttering.

What are the heart symptoms of Adonis vernalis?

It is a remedy which increases arterial tension, regulating the heart beat by lessening the frequency of the pulse and increasing the force of the cardiac contraction. The remedy is well tolerated; increases diuresis and acts with rapidity, otherwise the indications are the same as those of *Digitalis*. Its indications are rather physiological than homœopathic.

What are the heart symptoms of Convallaria?

Valvular diseases of the heart, with scanty urine and dropsy, and great dyspnœa. It is sometimes a useful remedy for dyspnœa, palpitation and œdema due to mitral disease.

What are the heart symptoms of Glonoine?

Fullness in region of heart, with some sharp pains; angina pectoris; fluttering of heart, with violent beating, as if chest would burst open; labored breathing.

Give symptoms of Naja tripudians in heart affections.

In valvular diseases of the heart, with a dry, teasing cough; there is tremulous action; it also acts on the left ovary, causing a pain there during the cough.

Give uses of Lycopus Virginicus in heart affections.

In cardiac irritability with depressed force, after abuse of cardiac depressants or of cardiac stimulants; excessive hypertrophy, muscular weakness, etc.

What are the indications for the use of Amyl nitrite?

In angina pectoris; during the attack there is oppressed breathing and constriction about the heart, and the slightest thing causes flushing.

Give heart symptoms of Ammonium carb.

Dilatation of the heart; patient suffers in a warm room and when ascending stairs or a height; palpitation; dyspnœa, retraction of the epigastrium; perhaps cyanosis.

When is Arnica a heart remedy?

Hypertrophy from heavy work; swelling of hands from any exertion; heart feels as if grasped; chest feels sore and bruised.

What remedies have a cold feeling about the heart?

Petroleum, *Nat. mur.*, *Graph.* and *Kali nitr.*

When is Lithium carb. indicated in heart affections?

Rheumatic soreness about heart; marked pain in heart when patient bends forward; shocks and jerks about heart; cardiac pains are relieved when patient urinates.

HERPES.

(See Skin, Diseases of.)

HOARSENESS.

Mention some remedies for the Hoarseness of singers.

Causticum, *Graphites*, *Selenium* and *Sulphur*.

How does the Hoarseness of Carbo veg. compare with that of Causticum?

It is aggravated in the evening, being useful after exposure to damp evening air, while *Causticum* is useful for hoarseness in dry, cold, severe winter weather, worse in the morning.

Give the indications for Phosphorus in Hoarseness.

Hoarseness worse in the evening, when it may be aphonia; great sensitiveness of the larynx; it hurts him to talk or cough; the voice is hoarse and rough.

Give the symptoms of Causticum in Hoarseness.

Complete loss of voice; the patient cannot speak loud; dryness of the larynx and sensitiveness extending to chest; there is a hoarseness, rawness, and a scraping sensation in the chest, especially under the middle of the sternum, giving rise to a dry and hollow cough.

How does Phosphorus differ?

Phosphorus has evening hoarseness, and the soreness of *Phosphorus* is in the larynx; while *Causticum* has morning hoarseness, soreness under the sternum, and a cough relieved by a cold drink.

Why should these two drugs especially be carefully differentiated?

Because they are inimical.

Compare also Eupatorium perf. with Causticum.

Both have hoarseness in the morning, both have influenza and aching in body, but *Eupatorium* has rather a chest soreness than a burning or rawness.

What drug has Aphonia from paretic state of laryngeal muscles?

Gelsemium.

Give some indications for Senega.

Hoarseness, and a throat so dry that it hurts to talk; great accumulation of albuminous mucus on the chest, which is difficult to expectorate. Great soreness of the chest.

Give indications for Argentum metallicum in affections of singers and speakers.

There is a copious exudation of mucus in the larynx; burning and rawness in the larynx, which is worse from talking or using the voice. The mucus is easily hawked up.

What characterizes the Hoarseness of Ammonium caust.?

Burning rawness in the throat; aphonia.

Give indications for Arum triph.

Hoarseness of singers and orators; voice suddenly gives out or suddenly breaks and goes to another key, from overuse of voice.

What remedies are useful for the Hoarseness of singers coming on as soon as they commence to sing?

Selenium and *Graphites*.

HYDROCEPHALUS.

In what disease is Helleborus most often called for and what are the indications?

Hydrocephalus; in stage of effusion; with signs of depression; stupor and unconsciousness; pupils sluggish; forehead corrugated, automatic action of one arm or one leg; the face flushes and pales; drinks greedily from nervousness; child suddenly screams out and bores its head into the pillow; the head is hot and the eyeballs are distorted; motion of jaws as if chewing.

Give indications for Apis in this affection.

Child bores its head backwards into the pillow, rolls it from side to side, rouses from sleep with a shrill, piercing cry; one side of the body may be convulsed or paralyzed; there is strabismus and the urine is scanty.

How does Apocynum compare here?

It is suitable to more advanced cases; the head is large, the fontanelles are wide open; it lacks the cephalic cry of *Apis*.

When should we choose Digitalis in Hydrocephalus?

When the urine is scanty and albuminous, and when the pulse is slow; perhaps cold sweat on surface of body.

When should Sulphur be given?

When *Apis* fails and when general *Sulphur* symptoms are present; the child is in a stupor; cold sweat, jerking of the limbs, suppressed urine; child wants to lie with its head low; cries out in sleep as if frightened; face red and pupils dilated.

HYSTERIA.

What are the indications for the use of Asafœtida in Hysteria?

Sensation of a ball rising from the stomach to the throat; worse from nervous excitement. There is a great deal of flatus, with oppressed breathing.

What is the applicability of Castoreum?

For nervous, irritable women, who do not react after severe diseases; women who are "pretty near" the hysterics.

What are the indications for Ignatia in Hysteria?

Great sensitiveness to external impressions, patients laugh and cry alternately, face flushes on emotion, spasmodic laughing ending in screaming, globus hystericus; profuse pale urine, flatulent conditions, contortions of the muscles. Clavus hystericus. Patient is hurried in her movements.

Give the symptoms indicating Moschus in Hysteria.

The patient faints from the least excitement; the hysterical spasm is ushered in by a contractive feeling about the throat; suffocation, globus hystericus; spasms about the chest and alternate crying and laughing.

Give the characteristic indications for Nux moschata.

Hysteria, with attacks of faintness and an irresistible desire to sleep; enormous bloating of the abdomen even after a slight meal and great dryness of the mouth; dyspepsia from any mental effort; distress appears while eating.

Give the general symptoms of the Tarentula Hispana.

Its chief characteristic is extreme restlessness; the patient must be in constant motion, though motion aggravates; must be doing something all the time; useful in hysterical affections.

Compare Valeriana in Hysteria.

It corresponds to general nervous and vascular excitement. Must keep constantly on the move. Slightest exertion causes headache and the slightest pain causes fainting; there are pains in the limbs, simulating rheumatism, which are better by walking about.

What are the hysterical symptoms in Platina?

The patient has a self-exaltation and self-esteem. Her laughter is loud and boisterous, and there is a marked mania.

What drugs have the globus hystericus?

Principally *Ignatia* and *Asafœtida*.

What is a remedy for headache in hysterical women which is caused by the slightest exertion?

Valerian.

Give some hysterical symptoms of Apis.

The patient is excitable, restless and fidgety. They are awkward and clumsy, and laugh in a silly way.

What other remedy has fidgets?

Zincum valeriana. They must keep feet and legs in constant motion.

INFLUENZA.

What would be the indications for Eupatorium perf. in Influenza or La Grippe?

Great soreness and aching of the entire body; hoarseness and cough, with great soreness of the larynx and chest; a great deal of coryza and thirst, and drinking causes vomiting; the cough hurts the head and chest and the patient holds the chest with the hands.

What other drug has this?

Drosera.

Give indications for Sabadilla.

Sneezing and lachrymation on going into open air; throat is swollen and pain is worse on empty swallowing. The sneezing is excessive and shakes the whole body.

When is Arsenicum iod. indicated?

Chills, with flushes of heat and severe fluent coryza; discharge irritating and corrosive; sneezing and prostration.

When is Gelsemium the remedy?

Patient is weak and tired; aching throughout the body; chilly, hugs the fire. Paroxysms of sneezing with excoriating discharge.

Give some characteristic indications for Dulcamara.

Suffused eyes, sore throat, cough hurts because of muscular soreness. Fever heat, and restlessness not specially pronounced.

INJURIES.

In what general condition is Arnica a remedy?

In mechanical injuries, sudden wrenching of muscles from strains, hemorrhages from injuries; for injuries to the soft parts accompanying fractures, bruises, ecchymoses; concussions of the brain and spine.

When, in injuries, is Rhus tox. preferable?

Where the ligaments rather than the soft parts are injured, for it acts more on the fibrous tissues.

When would Hypericum be indicated?

When there is injury to the nerves. It has been called the "Arnica of the nerves."

Give indications for Calendula in wounds.

When the wounds are ragged and there is loss of substance with great soreness and pain; it reduces inflammation and promotes healthy granulation.

When should Staphisagria be thought of?

In symptoms traceable to surgical operations, smooth, clean cuts, etc.

What is the remedy for injuries to bone?

Sympnytum off.

To what form of injury is Ledum suitable?

To punctured wounds or those made with pointed instruments.

What is the remedy for indurations remaining after injuries and for bruises of glands?

Conium.

What remedy is useful for long-lasting black and blue spots with soreness and stiffness?

Sulphuric acid.

What is a useful remedy for old sprains?

Ruta grav.

INSOMNIA.
(See Sleep, Affections of.)

INSANITY.
(See Mental Conditions and Derangements.)

INTERMITTENT FEVER.

Give indications for Arsenicum in Intermittent Fever.

The paroxysms are not complete, they are more apt to occur at night with sweat at the end of the fever; the thirst is never with the chill, it occurs after it; but during the sweat there is violent thirst, especially for hot drinks, since cold drinks chill; the pulse is small, frequent and weak.

What are the febrile symptoms of Apis?

Chill without thirst, followed by burning heat of the whole body and oppression of the chest, sweat partial without thirst; nettle rash.

What are the chill symptoms of Capsicum?

The chill commences in the back with thirst, but drinking causes shivering, associated with pain in the back and limbs.

What are the symptoms of Cinchona in Intermittent fever?

Restlessness before the chill, absence of thirst during chill and heat, but marked thirst during the sweat; during the chill wants to be covered, but has no relief therefrom; during heat wants to uncover, but becomes chilly on doing so; sweat is profuse and debilitating; yellow, sallow face; no characteristic time, perhaps occurring more in the afternoon and evening; all stages well marked, anticipating chill every second day. During apyrexia patient feels well (*Arsenic*, feels sick and miserable).

How does this differ from Chininum sulph. or the Sulphate of Quinine?

Here the chill returns with great regularity, clear intermissions, regular paroxysms, nearly clean tongue and profuse sweats.

When should Ipecac be given?

When the case is mixed up; there is a short chill, long fever, a predominence of gastric symptoms, and marked nausea.

Give indications for Cornus florida, another remedy useful in Intermittent Fever.

Sleepy before chill; dullness, drowsiness, headache and exhaustion; very weak between paroxysms, with diarrhœa and jaundiced skin.

What is the principal Homœopathic use of Eupatorium perfoliatum and its indications?

Intermittent fever. The chill commences about seven or nine in the morning, in the back, accompanied by thirst, and there is intense aching in all the bones, as if they were broken; this is followed by heat and an increase of the aching, and this by a scanty or profuse sweat.

Give a characteristic of the drug in these conditions that is even more characteristic than the break-bone pains.

It is the vomiting. The patient vomits water or food that has been taken, or of bile as the chill passes of.

What is the Chill of Ferrum?

It is a chill with red face and thirst; during the heat there is distention of the blood-vessels and headache; the chill is apt to come on about three or four in the morning.

What characterizes the Intermittent Fever of Gelsemium?

The chill runs up the back; there is aching all over the body; the patient wants to be held so that he won't shake so; noise and light are intolerable; sweat is partial, but it relieves all the pains; copious urination also relieves. The patient is characteristically drowsy, dull and dizzy; there is absence of thirst and great muscular soreness.

What is the Fever of Ignatia?

Partial in all its stages; the chill is not relieved by external heat, and there is thirst with the chill, but none with the fever.

What is the Fever of Natrum muriaticum?

It is useful in intermittent fever from living in damp regions, especially after the abuse of *Quinine;* the chill comes on in the morning at ten o'clock, preceded by headache, thirst, backache, and accompanied by fever blisters on the lips; there is also vomiting with the chill.

What are the febrile symptoms of Natrum sulphuricum?

It is a useful remedy in bilious intermittent fevers, accompanied by liver affections, jaundice and bilious diarrhœa.

Give the symptoms of Nux in Intermittent Fever.

Chill begins in the extremities, with blueness of nails; gaping and yawning, and aching in the limbs; thirst with the chill, not before it as in *China*, and as chill passes off the patient vomits; the fever is especially in the upper part of the body. Gastro-bilious symptoms predominate.

What is the characterizing indication for Rhus in Intermittent Fever?

A dry, teasing cough during the chill, and hydroa.

What are the symptoms calling for Carbo veg. in Intermittent Fever?

After abuse of *Quinine;* thirst during chill and coldness of legs up to the knees; the heat is in burning flashes; sweat is sour and offensive; during apyrexia, pale and weak.

Give the symptoms indicating Lachesis.

Chill in afternoon, one or two; during chill patient must have clothing piled on him, not so much to keep him warm as to keep him still; the heat is burning; there is oppression of the chest and drowsiness.

IRITIS.

(See Eye, Diseases of.)

KIDNEYS, DISEASES OF.

Give some indications for Arsenicum in Bright's Disease.

General anasarca, œdema and puffiness; albuminous urine; waxy casts; skin pale and waxy looking; exhausting diarrhœa; burning and thirst; frequent vomiting. The presence of blood boils is also an indication.

Give indications for Mercurius corrosivus in Kidney Disease.

The urine is thick, and micturition difficult; urine contains albumen, granular and fatty tube casts and epithelial cells; there is more or less inflammation at the neck of the bladder; face pale and swollen; pulse irregular and uneven.

Give indications for Digitalis in renal affections

Dropsy; feeble or slow pulse; scanty, dark, turbid urine, which is albuminous; similar to *Arsenic*, without its restlessness and irritability.

When is Apis indicated in Bright's Disease?

Urine scanty and albuminous; anasarca with white, shining skin; ascites, with soreness of abdominal walls.

What are the indications for Terebinth?

Pressure in kidneys while sitting; urine scanty, smoky and dark; much albumen and many bloody casts. Bloody urine is the keynote. The pain is burning and extends into right hip.

Give symptoms of Cantharis.

Aching across loins; albuminous, high colored urine, with scalding.

What are the renal symptoms of Berberis?

Deep and severe pains in region of the kidney, extending down back and along the uterus into the pelvis. Pains seem to radiate in all directions from the kidneys. Useful for renal calculi.

When is Phosphorus the remedy in Bright's Disease?

The urine contains epithelial, fatty or waxy casts; abuse of alcoholic stimulants, lung complications, vomiting or diarrhœa. Urine is whitish, flocculent, iridescent.

LABOR.

When should Chamomilla be given during Labor?

When the pains begin in the back and pass off down the inner side of the thighs, and when the patient is intolerant of the pain, makes a great fuss, is impatient and spiteful, the os being rigid.

What are the indications for Belladonna in Labor?

Pain in back as if it would break; labor pains come and go suddenly and no progress is made; there is a spasmodic condition of the os which retards labor; the os feels hot to the touch.

When is Secale indicated Homœopathically in Labor?

When the pains are prolonged, continued and ineffectual or entirely wanting, and patient complains of an empty feeling in the abdomen.

When should Caulophyllum be used during Labor?

When the pains are intermittent, sharp and crampy, and appear in the groin, bladder and lower extremities; they are spasmodic and fly from one place to another; patient is exhausted and weak.

What is another indication for its use in the puerperal state?

For false labor pains occurring during last months of pregnancy; after pains following a tedious labor.

What is the chief indication for Gelsemium in Labor?

Rigid os uteri from tardy dilatation; uterus soft and flabby; does not contract or expel; patient drowsy; premonitory stage of puerperal convulsions.

Where are the Labor pains of Cimicifuga?

They fly across the abdomen, from side to side; double patient up and cause fainting spells. Also for false labor pains shooting upwards and transversely; after pains.

How does Pulsatilla compare?

The pains are slow, weak and ineffectual; they are spasmodic and irregular and excite fainting; the temperament will decide, or the smothering sensation, that the patient has, calling for open windows. Adherent placenta.

LARYNGITIS.

Give the indications for Hepar in laryngeal affections.

The cough of *Hepar* is never a dry one, it has a slight *loose edge;* the expectoration is slight, and there is little fever. Croup, where the patient is sensitive to the least draft of air; it comes in here after *Aconite* and *Spongia*.

In acute Laryngitis when should Spongia be given?

Where the cough is harsh and barking, where there are suffocative spells during sleep with external sensitiveness to the touch.

What are laryngeal symptoms of Arum triphyllum?

Hoarseness and rawness in the larynx; the control over the voice is lost; the voice suddenly changes; dry cough; patient cringes under it, it hurts so.

What are the laryngeal symptoms of Argentum metallicum?

Hoarseness, rawness and burning in the larynx, and a copious exudation into the larynx; looking like boiled starch; it is easily expectorated; chronic hoarseness and soreness of the larynx; chronic laryngitis of singers and speakers.

Mention the most important remedies in Laryngismus stridulus.

Chlorine, Lach., Bell., Bromine, Gelsem. and *Sambucus.*

What are the main indications for Aconite in Laryngitis?

The fever, rough throat, hoarseness, sensitiveness to air and the thin, frothy expectoration.

Mention a serviceable adjuvant in the treatment of acute Laryngitis.

Inhalations of hot steam from an atomizer.

Mention three remedies useful in Œdema of the Glottis.

Arsenic, Apis and *Lachesis.*

LEUCORRHŒA.

What is the Leucorrhœa of Hydrastis?

Like all the secretions of *Hydrastis* it is thick, yellow and tenacious, and is accompanied with great weakness and constipation.

Give the Leucorrhœa of Alumina.

It is very ropy and tenacious, yellowish bland mucus, and exhausts very much, as it is rich in albumen.

When is Graphites indicated in Leucorrhœa?

When it is profuse and thin white mucus, comes in gushes, and is excoriating. Patients are constantly cold.

When is Aletris indicated?

When the leucorrhœa is associated with extreme constipation and weakness of digestion.

What is the Leucorrhœa of Pulsatilla?

Thick, yellowish, green and bland like all *Pulsatilla* discharges.

When is Calcarea phos. useful?

In leucorrhœa of little girls. Profuse, milky, purulent, with itching and burning.

What is the Leucorrhœa of Borax?

It is clear, copious and albuminous, and has an unnatural heat to it. It is acrid and occurs midway between the menstrual periods with swelling of labia.

What is the Leucorrhœa of Kreasote?

It is very acrid, irritating and excoriates the parts; it is profuse and watery. Yellowish leucorrhœa with great debility. Micturition painful.

Give Leucorrhœa of Calcarea carb

The leucorrhœa is burning and itching; worse before menses.

Give Leucorrhœa of Lilium tig

Watery, yellowish, yellowish-brown and excoriating.

When is Belladonna useful?

In thin, odorless, bland leucorrhœa, due to congestion of the uterus; it is increased by any cause producing pelvic congestion.

When is Helonias indicated?

Profuse, yellow leucorrhœa; thick, irritating, causing some itching. Patient is anæmic and sallow. Leucorrhœa aggravated by colds or overexertion.

What is the Leucorrhœa of Sepia?

Milky; worse before menses, with bearing down in pelvis. Patient is sallow, suffers from pimples, itching of the skin and headache.

When should Stannum be given?

Profuse, bland leucorrhœa, consisting of white or yellow mucus, accompanied with great debility. Patients are weak and have backache.

LIVER, DISEASES OF.

What is the action of Mercurius on the liver?

The skin and conjunctiva are jaundiced; the region of the liver is sore to the touch. The patient cannot lie on the right side. The liver is enlarged. The stools are either clay colored, from absence of bile, or yellowish-green, bilious stools, passed with a great deal of tenesmus. There is a yellowish, white-coated tongue, which takes the imprints of the teeth, and there is a fetid breath.

What are the symptoms of Leptandra in liver affections?

There is aching in the region of the liver and soreness. There is drowsiness and despondency, and a dark, black, pitchy diarrhœa, which is accompanied by colicky pain at the umbilicus; the tongue is coated yellow or black down the middle.

What is the distinction between Leptandra and Mercurius?

Mercurius has tenesmus after stool, while *Leptandra* has no tenesmus, but griping, colicky pains; and under *Leptandra* there is a great deal of aching in the posterior part of the liver.

What are the liver symptoms of Nux vomica?

It is one of the best remedies for liver affections in those who have abused alcoholic liquors or drastic purgatives. The liver is swollen and sensitive to the pressure of clothing, and there is much colic with these bilious troubles. Accompanying these liver symptoms there are always hemorrhoids. With *Nux vom.* the pains and tenesmus cease after stool.

What are the symptoms of Podophyllum in liver affections?

It is indicated in torpid or chronically congested liver. The liver is swollen and sensitive. The face and eyes are yellow; there is a bad taste in the mouth. The tongue is coated yellow or white. The bile may form gall stones. There is a loose, watery diarrhœa, or if constipation be present the stools are clay colored.

What drug is known as vegetable Mercury?

Podophyllum.

What drugs have the symptom that the tongue takes the imprint of the teeth?

Mercurius, Podophyllum, Yucca, Rhus and *Stramonium.*

Give the general liver symptoms of Lycopodium.

There is sensitiveness in the region of the liver and a feeling of tension there; there is a feeling as though a cord were tied about the waist; the bowels are usually constipated; there is pressure of gas in the intestines and a sensation of satiety after eating.

What are the symptoms of Bryonia in liver affections?

There is a congested and inflamed liver; there are sharp stitching pains under the shoulder blade and in the right side; there is a bitter taste in the mouth; the pains are worse from any motion, and better when lying on right side; jaundice from duodenal catarrh brought on by fit of anger.

What are the liver symptoms of Chelidonium?

There is soreness and stitching pains in the region of the liver; the keynote for this drug in hepatic diseases is a pain under the angle of the right shoulder blade; there is swelling of the liver, chilliness, fever, jaundice, yellow coated tongue, bitter taste, and a craving for acids and sour things, such as pickles and vinegar. The stools are profuse, bright yellow and diarrhœic. The stools may also be clayey.

How does Bryonia differ from Chelidonium here?

Only in the character of the stools, which are hard, dry and brown, or if loose, associated with a colic similar to that of *Colocynth*.

What are the liver symptoms of Myrica cerifera?

There is first despondency; also jaundice due to imperfect formation of bile in the liver, and not to any obstruction of its flow. There is a dull headache, worse in the morning. The eyes have a dirty, dingy, yellowish hue. The tongue is coated dirty yellow. The patient is weak and complains of muscular soreness and aching in the limbs.

Give the liver symptoms of Digitalis.

Digitalis has jaundice which is due, as under *Myrica*, to functional imperfections of the liver; drowsiness, bitter taste and the jaundice can usually be traced to heart affections. There is also soreness, enlargement and bruised feeling in the region of the liver.

What are the symptoms of Taraxacum in liver affections?

In the first place there is a mapped tongue and bitter taste in the mouth. Chilliness after eating and drinking, pain and soreness in the region of the liver and bilious diarrhœa.

Give indications for Chionanthus Virginica.

Bitter eructations, bilious vomiting, sore aching over the body. In uncomplicated jaundice it is a prominent remedy. Skin and eyes yellow.

What other drug has a mapped tongue?

Kali bichromicum.

What are the symptoms of Yucca in liver affections?

There is a pain going from the upper portion of the liver to the back and a bad taste in the mouth. The stools are diarrhœic and contain an excess of bile, accompanied with a great deal of flatulence. Sallow, yellow face and tongue taking imprints of teeth.

What drugs have biliousness following an attack of anger?

Chamomilla and *Bryonia.*

What are the liver symptoms of Berberis vulgaris?

There are sharp, stitching pains in the region of the liver, pains shooting down to the umbilicus; there are sticking pains under the borders of the false ribs, which indicate a presence of gall stones.

What remedies cause Atrophy of the Liver?

Laurocerasus and *Phosphorus.*

What are the symptoms of Phosphorus in liver affections?

It is usually in fatty degeneration of the liver with well-marked soreness and jaundice; the stools are grayish white. It is also useful for cirrhosis and atrophy of the liver. The jaundice is indicative of organic disease. It is also a useful remedy for malignant diseases of the liver.

Give the general symptoms of Magnesia muriatica.

The liver is enlarged and the pains are worse from lying down on the right side. It is a useful remedy for enlarged liver of children who are puny in growth; and here we have the characteristic crumbling stools which distinguishes it from *Mercurius*. Also in bilious diarrhœa headache; pain in right side; œdema of lower extremities.

Give some liver symptoms of Carduus marianus.

There is jaundice, headache and bitter taste and nausea, with vomiting of acid, green fluids. There is an uncomfortable fullness in the region of the liver. The stools are bilious and the urine is golden yellow. Sensitiveness of epigastrium and right hypochondrium,

Give the symptoms of Natrum sulphuricum in liver affections.

There is aching and cutting in the region of the liver. The liver is engorged, and the symptoms are worse lying on the left side. There is jaundice, bilious colic, vomiting of bile and bitter mucus.

Give the symptoms of Kali bichromicum in so-called biliousness.

The skin is yellow, sallow and covered with pimples; the whites of the eyes are yellow; the tongue is thick, broad and mapped; there is morning diarrhœa, watery stools, and tenesmus, especially after drinking beer.

What is the effect of Carbo vegetabilis on the Liver?

It causes a sluggish circulation and portal stasis, which produces enlarged veins in the lower extremities, hemorrhoids, etc.; the patient likes to sit with the feet upon the table, because it favors the circulation.

Give the action of Sulphur on the Liver.

It increases the flow of bile; there is also much pain and soreness of the liver.

Give indications for Aurum in Liver affections.

Swollen and cirrhosed liver, burning and cutting in right hypochondrium; ascites; grayish or ashy white stools, and mental condition of low-spiritedness.

To what forms of Jaundice is China suitable?

To those which arise from sexual excesses, abuse of alcohol and from loss of animal fluids.

LOCOMOTOR ATAXIA.

Give symptoms which would indicate Alumina in Locomotor Ataxia.

The patient cannot walk without staggering if his eyes are closed; he feels as if he were walking on cushions; there is creeping as if ants were crawling on his legs and back, the extremities go to sleep, the legs are numb, and there is a sensation as if there were a cobweb on the face; there is also much severe pain in the back.

When is Zincum the Remedy?

Intense fulgurating pains with twitchings of various muscles, great restlessness of the limbs and impotence.

And when Phosphorus?

Burning along spine with tingling and formication in the extremities, weakness and trembling of limbs on beginning to walk, patient stumbles, catches his toe on every obstacle; imperfect coördination.

Give symptoms calling for Plumbum.

Wasting of paralyzed parts; total loss of coördination. Anæsthesia and paralysis of the limbs; loss of sexual desire and impotence.

Give indications for Ammonium muriaticum.

Fulgurating pains, rending, tearing, painful jerks in the thighs, lower limbs and joints with a sensation of soreness.

What are the indications for Secale in Locomotor Ataxia?

Difficult staggering gait, even complete inability to walk, not from lack of power, but on account of a peculiar unfitness to perform light movements with the limbs and hands; contraction of lower limbs on account of which the patient staggers; trembling of limbs, sometimes with pain, formication of hands and feet, legs feel as of wood or padded; impotence.

Mention some other remedies useful in these fulgurating pains of Locomotor Ataxia.

Chamomilla, Colocynth, Ferrum, Kali carbonicum and *Lycopodium.*

Give Homœopathic indications for Argentum nitricum in this disease.

Legs weak, calves bruised, soreness in lumbo-sacral region; pain in small of back, worse when rising; trembling of the hands; cannot walk in the dark or with his eyes closed. Legs feel like wood, loss of pupillary reflexes and incontinence of urine.

Give symptoms of Kali brom.

Legs numb and tingle, also spine. Sexual appetite increased; cannot manage legs; patient melancholic.

LUMBAGO.

(See Backache.)

MAMMARY GLAND, AFFECTIONS OF.

Where do the Pains of Croton tiglium extend when child is nursing?

To the back.

What are the symptoms calling for Phytolacca in affections of the mammary gland?

When the breasts show a tendency to cake and suppuration threatens, pain goes from nipple all over body, and there is excessive flow of milk.

What other drug has nodosities in the female breast, and how is it distinguished from Phytolacca?

Conium, here there is stony hardness, and it is less

acute than *Phytolacca;* in *Conium* the breasts are exceedingly sensitive, cannot bear the touch of clothes, and walking or jarring is painful.

Mention two other remedies that have nodes in the breast.

Calcarea fluorica and *Silicea*.

What is a symptom calling for Phellandrium?

When the pain courses along the milk ducts when child is not nursing.

What is the action of Pulsatilla on the Mammary Gland?

It is indicated when mechanical irritation excites flow of milk. It is also indicated where the flow of milk is scanty or absent, and where the patient is gloomy and tearful.

Mention some other drugs useful in Abscess of the Mammary Gland.

Bryonia, Belladonna and *Phosphorus*.

MARASMUS.

Give indications for Calcarea phosphorica in defective nutrition or Marasmus.

Thin, emaciated children, predisposed to glandular and osseous diseases; large head and open fontanelles; the teeth develop tardily; there is curvature of the spine, it is so weak it cannot support the body; the neck is very slim; the child vomits persistently; there is a diarrhœa of green, slimy and undigested stools.

Give indications for Iodine in Marasmus.

Extreme hunger, but in spite of this the patient emaciates; the function of the glands is interfered with; there is great torpidity and sluggishness of the system.

What are the indications for Magnesia carbonica in Marasmus?

Puny, sickly children, in whom milk causes pain when taken into the stomach, and is vomited undigested; there are griping, colicky pains; the stools are sour and green as grass; the child is improperly nourished; its mouth is full of ulcers.

How is Calcarea carb. distinguished?

By the sweat on head, by the damp, cold ·feet, and by the swollen abdomen.

When is Hepar the remedy?

It stands between *Sulphur* and *Calcarea*. There is weakness of digestion. Diarrhœa, worse during day and after eating; stools undigested and sour. The whole body smells sour.

What are the indications for Natrum mur.?

Thin necked children with ravenous appetite, yet they grow thin; great thirst; a constant heat and dryness of the mouth and throat, which water relieves.

MEASLES.

When should Bryonia be given in Measles?

When the rash appears late, and when it is apt to run

a bulky course, and when inflammatory diseases of the chest accompany. Dry, hard, painful cough.

What are the indications for Gelsemium in Measles?

The catarrhal symptoms, great prostration, stupor and absence of thirst; itching and redness of the skin.

Give indications for Aconite.

Best remedy at commencement; fever, restlessness, photophobia, coryza, sneezing and hard, croupy cough will indicate it.

What are three remedies for non-appearance or repercussion of the rash?

Stramonium. Child cries out, frightened, is convulsed, has bright red face.

Cuprum. Bluish face, violent symptoms, convulsive cramps, etc.

Zincum. Cries out in sleep; too debilitated to develop an eruption.

Give symptoms calling for Pulsatilla in Measles.

Coryza and profuse lachrymation. Cough dry at night, loose by day; child sits up to cough. Not in first stage of disease.

When does Kali bich. come in?

After *Pulsatilla*, with pustules on cornea; swelling of glands; shootings from ears into glands. Diarrhœa; symptoms in general are worse than those calling for *Pulsatilla*.

MENINGITIS.

When is Aconite the remedy in Meningitis?

When caused by exposure to the sun.

When is Apis the remedy?

The case is apt to commence with fidgetiness, there are shrill outcries in sleep. The eruption is either suppressed or undeveloped; stage of effusion. Squinting, grinding of teeth, violent fever.

Give in brief the indications for Belladonna.

The symptoms are severe and violent. There is intense congestion, throbbing, grinding of teeth and crying out in sleep; it pictures acute meningitis before exudation. Sharp pains, red face and acuteness of symptoms will call for this remedy.

When does Bryonia come in?

In the stage of effusion. Face flushes and pales alternately; child screams if moved the least. Has a hastiness in manner. White tongue and is thirsty.

Give indications for Cuprum in Meningitis.

When it arises from a suppressed eruption. There is violent delirium, blue face, convulsions, with clenched hands, rolling of eyeballs, grinding of teeth, followed by deep sleep.

What are the indications for Helleborus?

Stage of exudation. Shooting pains in head; bores

head into pillow; automatic motion of an arm and foot; eyeballs turned upwards; is hasty in manner.

Give indications for Zincum.

Sharp pains through head; especially in meningitis arising from non-development of an eruption; constant fidgety motions of feet. Little or no fever, and hyperæsthesia of all the senses and skin.

What remedies are useful in Tubercular Meningitis?

Artemesia vulgaris, *Baryta carb.* and *Calcarea carb.*

MENSTRUATION.

(See Women, Diseases of.)

MENTAL CONDITIONS AND DERANGEMENTS.

What are the mental symptoms of Aconite?

There is extreme restlessness, anxiety, tossing about and fear of death, even predicting the hour of death. There is an intolerance of music and there is a peculiar aversion to busy streets.

What other drug has the symptom that the patient predicts the hour of death?

Coffea.

What are the mental symptoms of Belladonna?

There is mental irritability, hasty speech and hasty action. There is a great deal of delirium. The patient desires to escape. He strikes those about him and tries to get out of bed. There is a desire to cut and tear the clothing, and is associated with a red face, throbbing carotids.

Veratrum album has almost the same symptoms. How is it distinguished from Belladonna?

There is coldness of surface of the body under *Verat. album* and cold sweat on forehead.

What other drugs have hasty speech and hasty drinking?

Lachesis and *Dulcamara* and *Sulphur*.

Give, in general, the mental symptoms of Hyoscyamus.

The patient is full of imaginations. Thinks he is about to be poisoned and refuses to take the medicine, and imagines that he is pursued by some one who is trying to take his life. The patient talks and mutters all the time, and jumps from one subject to another. There is delirium with involuntary passages and picking at the bed clothes and objects in the air. It is also a remedy for jealousy. Nymphomania, patient makes lewd gestures, throws off bed clothes, uncovers genitals.

What other drug has jealousy and great loquacity, the patient jumping from one subject to another?

Lachesis.

What are the mental symptoms of Stramonium?

There is wild delirium and a bright red face. The eyes have a suffused and wild look. The hallucinations terrify the patient; objects jump up from every corner; he sees all sorts of animals. At one moment he is laughing, singing and making faces and at another praying. There is constant loquacity, the talk being foolish and nonsensical. There is fear of the dark. He imagines that he hears voices. During delirium there are frequent attempts to escape. Bright objects cause delirium and spasms.

How is Stramonium distinguished from Lachesis in loquacity?

The *Stramonium* patient does not jump from one subject to another, but talks continually and foolishly, and it is distinguished also by the red face and other signs of sensorial excitement.

What drug causes a garrulity very much like that caused by tea, a sort of vivacity with love of prattling?

Paris quadrifolia.

What are the mental symptoms of Lachesis?

Loquacity, patient jumps from one subject to another; jealousy and a low muttering delirium with tendency of the lower jaw to drop, the patient being worse on waking; the mind is weakened; the patient thinks only with difficulty; ideas also crowd upon the mind rapidly; the patient thinks that he is under the control of some superhuman power.

What drug has the symptom that the patient thinks he has two wills, one commanding him to do what the other forbids?

Anacardium.

What other symptoms has Anacardium?

It produces a weak memory; he imagines he hears voices, and another condition is a propensity to swear; it is a mental condition and it does not exist as a result of low morals. The patient is also suspicious.

What other drug produces a disposition to swear?

Nitric acid.

What are the mental symptoms of Nux vomica?

The patient is irritable and ugly, easily put out; over-taxing of the mental powers aggravate the symptoms; disinclination to mental work; useful in over-worked, fidgety business men of sedentary habits.

What are the mental symptoms of Bryonia?

It is a useful remedy for abdominal symptoms resulting from fits of anger; the patient is irritable and easily angered; delirium in which the patient thinks he is away from home and wants to go home; talks about his business.

What are the mental symptoms of Chamomilla?

There is a peculiar excitability; the patient is cross and excitable, and slight impressions produce mental anguish; pains often result in fainting; it is a remedy for the effect of anger; children want to be carried about, and want different things, and when they get them throw them away dissatisfied; especially sensitive to pain, snappish, uncivil.

What drug has colic in children following fits of anger?

Staphisagria.

What are some other mental symptoms of Staphisagria?

It is a remedy for the affections of suppressed indignation. There is a hypochondriacal condition; the patient is apathetic and gloomy; he prefers solitude and is shy of the opposite sex. The *Staphisagria* child is impetuous and irritable, reminding one of *Chamomilla*.

What other drug is closely allied to both Chamomilla and Staphisagria in the bad effects of anger?

Colocynth.

What drugs, like Chamomilla, produce fainting from pains?

Valerian, Hepar sulphur and *Veratrum album.*

Give the mental symptoms of Aurum.

There is melancholy, with disposition to weep; feeling as if he were not fit to live, and a consequent tendency to suicide; often there is a religious mania; he prays all the time; the mind is full of suicidal thoughts; contradiction or dispute excites the patient, and there is great weakness of the memory; patient thinks he is damned.

What are the mental symptoms of Sepia?

The patient is low-spirited, cries readily; weak memory; there is sadness and irritability; it will not do to find fault with her; there is also perfect indifference, especially to household affairs and to her own family; the patient is easily offended; she dreads to be alone, wants company, but has an aversion to her own friends.

How is Sepia distinguished from Pulsatilla?

Both have weeping, anxiety, peevishness, and are ill-humored; but *Pulsatilla*, only, has the mild, clinging disposition calling for consolation; she makes her grief known and seeks sympathy. The *Sepia* patient is worse from gentle exercise, but is relieved by violent exercise.

How does Ignatia differ from both Pulsatilla and Sepia?

There is a tearful mood with melancholy under *Ignatia*, but the patients nurse their sorrows, and keep them from others.

Give some other mental symptoms of Ignatia.

It is especially a remedy for the effects of grief, particularly if the patient dwells upon her sorrows in secret, and especially if the cause of the grief be recent; changeable mood; introspective, given to sighing, full of disappointments; weeping.

What drug is useful for chronic or long-lasting effects of grief?

Phosphoric acid.

What are some mental symptoms of Phosphoric acid?

There is great indifference and torpidity of mind; the patient is disinclined to answer questions; he is in a stupor, unconscious of all that goes on around him, but when roused he is fully conscious; it is also a remedy for home-sickness; the patient is ill from the effects of grief.

Give some of the mental symptoms that would indicate Ignatia in hysteria.

The patient alternately laughs and cries, and there is great sensitiveness to external impressions; changeableness is characteristic; the patient sighs a great deal.

What are the mental symptoms of Platina?

The patient is proud and haughty; looks down upon others with disdain; everybody seems beneath her; objects seem unfamiliar to her—even familiar objects; she does not know where she is; there is often with this a condition of vision in which objects really look smaller; there is a great dread of death, which the patient believes to be near at hand. The proud, haughty feeling is the main characteristic.

What are the mental symptoms of Lycopodium?

The patient is impatient and irritable, gets angered easily and is apt to be domineering; at other times there is sadness and tearfulness; the memory is weak; they make mistakes in speech and forget words or syllables; afraid to be left alone.

What other drugs have the symptom that the patient has to think how words are spelled?

Sulphur and *Lachesis*.

What are the mental symptoms of Sulphur?

The patient has insane ideas; thinks she is wealthy; tears up her clothes and plays with old rags with pleasure, thinking that they are objects of beauty; there is also melancholy and restlessness; there is also a religious mania; patient fears she will not be saved; there is anxiety about her own soul, but perfectly indifferent about the souls of others; children are apt to be irritable and peevish,

What are the mental symptoms of Hepar sulph.?

The patient is low-spirited, and at times there is a tendency to suicide; the patient feels discouraged and cross, and annoyed by the recollection of past unpleasantnesses in his life; the memory is weakened; he forgets words or localities; he is over-sensitive, and speech is hasty; he is especially sad in the evening, and does not wish to see members of his own family.

What are the mental symptoms of Calcarea carbonica?

There is one peculiar symptom: the patients see persons and objects on closing the eyes; these disappear as soon as the eyes are open; there is an apprehensive state of the mind and fear that the patient will go crazy.

What other drugs have the first of these symptoms?

Belladonna and *Cinchona*.

What drugs have the symptom that the patient fears that he will go crazy?

Alumina and *Iodine*.

What are some of the other symptoms of Alumina?

The patient is low-spirited and inclined to weep, and there is a suicidal tendency when the patient sees blood or a knife. Then there is hypochondriasis and indifference to work; time passes slowly.

What mental symptoms call for Cannabis Indica?

There are great delusions as to time and distances. Time and space seem greatly extended. Objects a few feet off appear many yards away and seconds seem like a century.

What are the mental conditions of Apis?

The patient feels strange, as if about to die, but there is no fear of death. There is delirium and the mind is weak, but especially is there awkwardness. Patients let fall what they are carrying and run against furniture, etc., in a clumsy, awkward way.

What are the mental symptoms of Arsenic?

Here we have great fear of death also. There is great restlessness and desire to change position. They do not want to be left alone for fear they will die. The patient has fear of ghosts and fanciful figures.

How does the restlessness of Rhus tox. differ?

It is to relieve pain, not an anxious restlessness.

What are the mental symptoms of Natrum muriaticum?

The patient is sad and tearful. There is a low, depressed condition of the mind. The patient is worse from consolation. There is an intense degree of hypochodriasis. Then, too, the patient is irritable; every little trifle angers him, and unpleasant events trouble his mind and keep him awake. This melancholic condition is apt to follow excitement.

How does Natrum muriaticum differ from Pulsatilla in this tearful disposition?

Consolation under *Natrum mur.* aggravates, while under *Pulsatilla* the patient seeks consolation.

What drugs are useful for the bad effects of fright?

Opium, *Gelsemium*, *Pulsatilla* and *Veratrum album*.

What drugs are useful for chronic effects of fright?

Natrum mur., *Silicea* and *Phosphoric acid*.

Give the mental symptoms of Palladium.

The patient is easily put out of humor. Imagines herself neglected. Is proud, but the pride is easily wounded. She suffers from mental excitement, especially in company. Her symptoms are worse after an evening's excitement.

What are the mental symptoms of Antimonium crudum?

The children are cross and peevish; will not allow anyone to look at them. Adults are sulky and sad. In children this crossness is increased by washing them in water.

What are the mental symptoms of Gelsemium?

There is a tremor of the body and a great desire to be held still, and it is also a useful remedy for children after a fright. The patient is apathetic; does not seem to care "whether school keeps or not." Ailments from emotional excitement, such as bad news, fright, grief, etc.

Give the mental symptoms of Graphites.

The patient is full of grief, anxious and apprehensive, and this apprehensiveness compels her to move about from place to place. Has forebodings of accidents or mishaps which are about to take place. This makes her anxious and restless and she cannot keep still.

What is the Graphites temperament in general?

Sad, fat, fair and constipated.

What is the peculiar mental symptom of Argentum nitricum?

There is a sensation as if parts of the body were enormously large. The patient is impulsive, always busy yet accomplishes nothing. He makes mistakes in estimating distances. He is full of apprehension that he has some disease of the brain.

What are the peculiar mental symptoms of Baptisia?

There is a fear of being poisoned. The patient imagines that his body is scattered about in different places and that he has to move himself to get them together. There is a sensation as if the body were double or triple or scattered about in the bed; an indicative symptom to be found in typhoid fever.

What drug has the symptoms that the patient imagines herself double or that she is glass and is in constant fear of being touched lest she be broken?

Thuja.

What drugs have the sensation as though something were alive in the abdomen?

Thuja and *Crocus sativa.*

What other drugs have the symptoms besides Baptisia that the body is scattered about and the patient tries to get the pieces together?

Petroleum and *Thuja.*

What are the mental symptoms of Phosphorus?

The patient is susceptible to external impressions; can neither bear light, sounds nor odors; he is easily angered; has fanciful notions; sees faces in every part of the room, and all symptoms are aggravated by mental exertion; thoughts rush through his mind or else he has inability to think and remember.

What are the mental symptoms of Causticum?

The patient is low-spirited, nervous and anxious and fanciful; feels as though something were going to happen or as if he were going to commit a crime; it is also a remedy for the remote effects of anger; there is sadness, especially before the menses; she dreads the possibility of accidents to herself and others; afraid to go to bed in the dark.

What are the mental symptoms of Coffea?

It produces an ecstatic state of mind; unusual activity of mind and body; full of fancies; acuteness of all senses; great flow of thought.

What drug has the symptom that children wake at night unnaturally bright and playful, evincing no desire to go to sleep again?

Cypripedium.

What are the mental conditions of Glonoine?

There is forgetfulness; the patient loses her way in well-known streets; confusion of place.

What are the mental symptoms of Iodine?

There is a great dread of people; he shuns every one; the patient is excitable and restless, moves about from place to place.

What are the mental symptoms of Kali bromatum?

There are strange imaginations; the patient imagines that he will be poisoned; that he is hated by everybody. He will often imagine that he is pursued by some demon and will try to commit suicide to avert danger; there is also fear of being poisoned.

What are the mental symptoms of Kali carb.?

The patient is peevish and nervous and easily startled; imagines that someone is in the room; this anxiety is excited by any noise, such as shutting of a door or a window, and it sends them into a violent fit of trembling; there is great indifference; the patient does not know what she wants, and this condition is associated with great bodily exhaustion.

What are the mental symptoms of Lilium tigrinum?

There is a depressed mood; fears she will go crazy, and the patient feels relieved by diverting her mind or busying herself.

Mention two important drugs in home-sickness.

Pulsatilla and *Mercurius*.

What are the mental symptoms of Nux moschata?

There is a changeful mood; the patient laughs and jests about serious subjects, and then she changes to sadness, weeping and low crying; objects seem to grow smaller as she looks at them; there are errors in perception; bewilderment; there is a fanciful condition of the mind.

What are the mental conditions of Rhus tox?

There is delirium and restlessness; patient is indifferent; he fears that he will be poisoned and will not take the medicine on that account; there may be a desire to jump out of bed and try to escape, but it is not common.

What drug has a great deal of depression referable to the chest, is tearful and discouraged, and fears that he will go into decline?

Stannum.

What drug has the symptom that the soul feels as though it were free from the body?

Anacardium.

What drug has the symptom that patient fears that he will be run over in the street?

Phosphorus.

What are the mental conditions calling for the use of Kali phos.?

There is a gloomy, depressed irritable mental state; trifles annoy; the patient looks on the dark side of everything; there is a loss of memory, crossness and fretfulness in children.

What mental disease is Kali phos. useful in?

Melancholia and mania; somnambulistic states, or any state where there is mental aberration; hallucinations and illusions, puerperal mania and delirium tremens.

What are the mental symptoms of Natrum carbonicum?

Depressed and irritable, especially after a meal; this hypochondriasis decreases as the food gets out of the stomach into the bowels.

Give mental symptoms of Cimicifuga.

Mental depression; delirium tremens; visions of rats, mice, etc. A sensation as if there were a pall or gloom, or a horrible sadness settling over her—a feeling as if she were going crazy.

What are the mental symptoms of Cina?

The child wakes in a fright, screams, trembles and cannot be quieted; they are proof against all caresses; they are cross, irritable, nervous and peevish; they want to be rocked.

What is the mental condition of the Digitalis patient in heart affections calling for that remedy?

Anxious, low-spirited, gloomy and apprehensive, and a desire to be alone.

What are the mental symptoms of Conium?

Mental depression, hypochondriasis and hysteria, dread of society and of being alone.

What are the mental symptoms of Ambra?

Forgetfulness and hurry; the patient does everything in a hurry; time passes slowly.

What mental conditions has Colocynth?

Disturbances caused by mental emotions, violent anger or fright, vexation or mortified feelings.

What is the mental condition of the Pulsatilla patient?

A changeable disposition; first mild, tearful and yielding, and then irritable and peevish.

MISCARRIAGE.

What symptoms indicate Sabina?

Threatened abortion about the third month, with pains in the small of the back, going down thighs; bruised sensation along the anterior surface of the thighs. Pains running from sacrum to pubis is also a characteristic symptom.

What are the indications for Viburnum opulus?

Threatened miscarriage, with pains from lower abdomen into thighs.

When should Cimicifuga be thought of?

When the pains fly across the abdomen, from side to side, doubling the patient up; fainting spells.

What is an indication for the local use of Hamamelis in threatened Miscarriage?

Great soreness in the abdomen.

What drugs may be useful in threatened Miscarriage from anger?

Aconite and *Chamomilla*.

When is Secale indicated?

Threatened abortion during the later months; copious flow of black liquid blood, especially if the patient be thin and scrawny.

MOUTH, DISEASES OF.

What is the character of the sore mouth of Borax?

Aphthæ form on the inside of the cheeks, on the tongue and in the fauces; the mouth is hot; the membrane around these aphthæ bleeds easily, and the child lets go of the nipple and cries with vexation or refuses to nurse.

When is Mercurius indicated in this condition?

When there is salivation; the water dribbles from the child's mouth; diarrhœa with tenesmus.

What is a symptom of Bryonia which is sometimes useful in sore mouth?

The child refuses to nurse until mouth has been moistened, the mouth is so dry.

Give symptoms indicating Baptisia in affections of the mouth.

Fetor, salivation. Stomacace in last stages of phthisis.

When is Nitric acid indicated?

Pricking pains in mouth; aphthæ; gums whitish.

And Muriatic acid?

Deep ulcers with dark edges. Mucous membrane denuded and dotted with aphthæ.

Give indications for Arsenicum in sore mouth.

Burning in mouth; gangrene of the mouth; bluish or black sloughing ulcers. Gums bleed, tongue blistered.

Mention some remedies for common canker sores.

Lycopodium, when near frænum of the tongue.
Lachesis when at tip of the tongue.
Nitric acid, *Phytolacca* and *Natrum hydrochlor.* when on inner side of cheeks.
Salicylic acid, with burning soreness and fetid breath.

MUMPS.

In what diseases about the throat is Rhus tox. often indicated?

Mumps or swelling of parotid glands, with sticking pains when swallowing; they are dark red and worse on the left side.

When is Pulsatilla indicated?

When there is a threatened metastasis to the breasts or testicles.

Give indications for Belladonna.

Bright red swelling, especially on right side, or where the swelling suddenly disappears and cerebral symptoms ensue.

What are the indications for Mercurius?

Swelling is pale; the jaws are stiff; much pain and salivation.

NEURALGIA.

When should Aconite be given in Neuralgia?

When there is violent congestion of the parts, and they are hot and swollen; when brought on by exposure to dry, cold winds; and where the pains are tingling and drive the patient to despair; also with numb sensations. Pains worse at night.

What neuralgic symptoms has Allium cepa?

Neuralgias following amputations, and injuries of nerves with fine, shooting, thread-like pains; neuralgia of stumps.

What other remedy has neuralgic pains in stumps?

Ammonium mur.

What are the symptoms of Arsenicum in Facial Neuralgia?

Fine pains course through the face like burning needles; the face is pale and shrunken. Malarial neuralgias.

What are the nervous symptoms of Belladonna?

Neuralgic pains, which come on suddenly and disappear suddenly; lancinating pains, aggravated by motion. Convulsions and spasms in teething children, from repelled eruption, with red face, hot head, throbbing carotids, starting from sleep in terror.

What is the main use of Cedron?

Neuralgias, which return with clock-like periodicity; supra-orbital neuralgias or chills of malarial origin, which are regular as a clock.

When is Cinchona indicated in Neuralgia?

Periodical infra-orbital neuralgias of malarial origin, where the slightest draft makes the patient worse.

What are the neuralgic symptoms of Mezereum?

Neuralgia of cheek bones with numbness; neuralgic pains along an eruption as in herpes zoster; ciliary neuralgias.

What are the indications for Spigelia in Facial Neuralgia?

The pains are severe, sticking and burning, and the parts swell and become very sore. It occurs more on the left side.

How is it to be distinguished from Colchicum?

In *Spigelia* there is great nervous erethism and excitement and intolerance of pain, while in *Colchicum* there is a remarkable tolerance of pain with a general semi-paralytic condition, instead of nervous excitement.

Differentiate briefly between Spigelia and Arsenic, Platina, Chamomilla, Capsicum and Verbascum in Facial Neuralgia

Arsenic. Fine, red-hot, needle-like pains darting from place to place.

Platina. Steady compression, with numbness, wants to rub the part.

Chamomilla. Great impatience and aggravation by heat.

Capsicum. Fine lines of pain; worse from external pressure.

Verbascum. Pains are crushing, as if parts were between tongs, while under *Spigelia* the pains are shooting and piercing and the chief seat is about the eye.

What are the neuralgic symptoms of Stannum?

The guiding symptom to its use in neuralgia is that the pains increase and decrease gradually.

What are the Neuralgias and peculiar symptoms about the head found under Thuja?

Sensation as though a nail were being driven into the vertex or frontal eminences, intense stabbing pains driving patient almost to distraction; patient must lie down.

What are the Neuralgias of Cimicifuga?

They are mostly reflex from ovarian or uterine disease.

Mention two other drugs useful for Neuralgia with burning pains.

Kalmia and *Kreasote*.

Give indications for Magnesia.

The principal indication calling for this remedy is relief from warm applications.

NEURASTHENIA.

Give indications for Picric acid in Neurasthenia.

Depression and weariness from slight fatigue, a mental inactivity with indifference and a desire to lie down and rest; brain fag; the grand characteristic is that the slightest exertion brings on speedy exhaustion, and extinguishes that quality which we call *grit*.

What symptoms call for Phosphoric acid?

Exhaustion from over-work; heaviness in head and limbs; vertigo, formication in back, legs weak.

When is Silicea indicated?

Patient dreads exertion of body or mind; numbness of fingers, toes and back.

Give symptoms of Zincum.

Backache, worse while sitting ; burning in spine; weak limbs; formication in calves.

When is Phosphorus indicated?

Sudden prostration ; the nervous system seems to have sustained a sudden shock.

ŒDEMA OF GLOTTIS.

(See Laryngitis.)

OPHTHALMIAS.

(See Eye, Diseases of.)

ORCHITIS.

What symptoms would call for Clematis?

In orchitis, when it is of gonorrhœal origin, and when the testicle is indurated and hard as a stone and very painful.

Compare it with Rhododendron.

In *Rhododendron* the testicle tends to atrophy; there is a crushed feeling in the gland, and it is more useful in chronic cases; both drugs have pains which course up the spermatic cord.

What are the principal affections about the male sexual organs calling for Pulsatilla?

Orchitis and epididymitis, where the testicle is retracted, enlarged, sensitive and dark red, with pains along the spermatic cord, especially when due to suppression of a gonorrhœal discharge.

Mention four drugs that should be compared with Pulsatilla in swelled testicles.

Rhododendron, Clematis, Iodine and *Spongia*.

What are the symptoms of Rhododendron in Orchitis?

Hard, indurated testicle, with tendency to atrophy and a sensation as if it were crushed; drawing in spermatic cord, extending to abdomen and thigh.

Give the indications for Spongia in Orchitis.

Where there is hardness and squeezing pains in the testicles and cord, worse from any motion; great enlargement of the testicles.

Mention a remedy useful in chronic Orchitis.

Aurum.

What remedy is indicated in swelled testicles by the exquisite soreness of the parts.

Hamamelis.

OTITIS.

(See Ear, Diseases of.)

OVARIAN DISEASES.

What are the symptoms indicating Apis in ovarian troubles?

It affects especially the right ovary. Ovaritis with soreness in the inguinal region, with burning and stinging and tumefaction. Ovarian cysts in their incipiency; numbness down the thigh; tightness across the chest or a reflex cough accompany.

What are indications for Belladonna in Ovaritis?

Acute ovaritis, especially if the peritoneum be involved, with clutching, throbbing pains. If on the right side the drug will be more indicated. Great sensitiveness, the slightest jar unbearable.

What are the ovarian symptoms of Graphites?

Swelling and induration of left ovary.

Give indications for Lachesis in ovarian troubles.

Pain in the left ovary relieved by a discharge from the uterus; can bear nothing heavy on this region.

Give the ovarian symptoms for Platina.

The ovaries are sensitive and have burning pains in them.

Give symptoms of Argentum metallicum.

Affects left ovary, causing bruised pain and sensation as if ovary were growing large.

Give ovarian symptoms of Arsenicum?

Affects more right ovary; there is burning, tensive pains in the ovaries, but there must be evidences of ovaritis present; hot applications relieve.

When is Palladium indicated?

Swelling and induration of right ovary.

Mention a remedy useful for ovarian colic, where it is relieved by bending double.

Colocynth.

OZÆNA.

(See Catarrhal Troubles.)

PARALYSIS.

What are the symptoms of Causticum about the face, mouth and throat?

There is paralysis of the face, due to exposure to dry, cold winds; there is also a paralysis of the tongue, lips and throat.

How does Aconite compare here?

Like *Causticum* it has paralysis due to dry, cold winds, but it is more suitable to the beginning, *Causticum* coming in after *Aconite* fails.

What is the effect of Dulcamara on the nervous system?

Paralysis from lying on the damp ground; paralysis of the bladder or of any part of the body which is brought on or made worse by damp weather.

Give some of the nervous disturbances of Gelsemium.

Loss of power of muscular control, cramp in muscles of forearm; professional neurosis, such as writers' cramp, violin players' cramp, etc. Excessive trembling of all limbs, ptosis and other paralyses, post diphtheritic paralyses.

What are the paralytic symptoms of Plumbum?

Paralysis of the extensor muscles of the wrist, wrist drop; the paralysis is accompanied by atrophy of the affected parts, or they suffer from fatty degeneration.

Mention two drugs useful in paralysis of the bladder?

Dulcamara and *Hepar*.

Give paralytic symptoms of Rhus tox.

Paralysis of any part in rheumatic subjects as a result of getting wet; chronic cases.

Mention some remedies having ptosis or paralysis of the upper eyelid.

Rhus, Sepia, Kalmia, Causticum and *Gelsemium*.

What are the indications for Zincum?

Paralysis from cerebral softening, from suppressed foot sweat; there is vertigo, trembling, numbness and formication.

PAROTITIS.
(See Mumps.)

PERITONITIS.

What are the indications for Belladonna in Peritonitis and inflammation about the abdomen?

Swollen, tense, sensitive abdomen, cannot bear the weight of the bed clothes, jarring of the bed aggravates, on raising the clothes the heat streams out.

Give indications for Bryonia.

There must be present the sharp stitching pains and the aggravation from motion; there may or may not be high fever.

Give symptoms calling for Arsenicum.

Sudden sinking of strength; restlessness and thirst; constant vomiting and burning in abdomen; copious and persistent exudation.

PHTHISIS.

What are the special indications for Arsenicum iodatum in tubercular conditions?

The great debility, the night sweats and the decided cachectic appearance of the patient, the recurring fever, the emaciation, the profound prostration and the tendency to diarrhœa.

Give some indications for Calcarea phosphorica in Phthisis.

Associated with fistula in ano; chronic cough, with cold extremities; profuse night sweats in phthisis; sweat, especially about the head and neck. Incipient phthisis in anæmic subjects.

What are the indications for Nitric acid in Phthisis?

Difficult, green, purulent expectoration; night sweats; soreness of the chest; hectic; hemorrhages; dyspnœa and hoarseness, worse in the morning.

Compare Calcarea carb. here.

Pale, light complexion, painless hoarseness; the chest soreness is worse from touch or pressure; dyspnœa and loose, rattling cough are the characteristics of *Calcarea;* while thin, dark complexion, stinging hoarseness, chest soreness, not worse from touch or pressure, palpitation and intermittent pains on going up stairs, morning diarrhœa and tight dry cough are the characteristics of *Nitric acid*.

Give some further symptoms of Calcarea calling for its use in Phthisis.

Pain in the right side of the chest; mucous rales which are worse on the right side; purulent expectoration; great emaciation and sweat; there is great shortness of breath, especially on going up stairs; there is dry cough at night, and it is apt to be loose during the day; the expectoration tastes sweetish.

Give an indication for Tuberculinum.

Tubercular troubles, tubercular meningitis, consumption or tubercular arthritis. Dr. Burnett reports several cures of phthisis with *Bacillinum*, which is practically the same as *Tuberculinum*. Constant disposition to catch cold.

Give the indication for Sulphur in Tuberculosis.

In the beginning of the disease, with pain through the left chest, heat on the head, cold feet, frequent flushes, the patient wanting the window open.

Is Spongia ever indicated in Phthisis pulmonalis; if so, with what symptoms?

Hard, ringing, metallic cough, worse from deep breathing, with a sensation of weakness as if the patient would fall, worse from deep breathing, talking and dry, cold winds; flashes of heat which return when thinking of them.

Differentiate Carbo animalis from Carbo vegetabilis in Phthisis.

Carbo an. has hoarse cough; sensation as if brain were loose; green, purulent and offensive expectoration; when patient closes his eyes sensation of smothering.

Carbo veg. Deep spasmodic cough, with smothering burning in chest; profuse yellow expectoration, more fetid than that of *Carbo animalis;* there is dyspnœa and rattling in chest.

Give the chest symptoms of Stannum.

A teasing cough which is worse at night, with shortness of breath, profuse sweats, and great weakness; the expectoration tastes sweetish and is of a light yellow or lemon color; this is characteristic.

When is Silicea indicated in Phthisis?

Cough increased by rapid motion; copious rattling of mucus in chest; expectoration purulent; catarrhal phthisis of old people.

How do Phosphorus and Stannum compare?

Both have hectic, copious sputa, evening aggravation, hoarseness, etc., but *Phosphorus* has more blood streaks and more oppression of chest.

What is another drug that has been used clinically for copious purulent expectoration?

Balsam Peru.

What are two remedies for the dry, teasing night coughs of Phthisical patients?

Codeine and *Laurocerasus.*

Give symptoms calling for Sanguinaria.

Hectic fever; cheeks have a bright, circumscribed flush; cough is dry; there is burning and fullness in the chest and sharp pains in right lung, and dyspnœa.

Give the respiratory symptoms of Arsenicum.

Great dyspnœa, with restlessness and exhaustion; cough dry, fatiguing and whistling, with sensation as of fumes of sulphur in the larynx; rawness, soreness, and dryness, and burning in the chest; cough worse after midnight.

What drug has a dry cough worse before midnight?

Sulphur.

PLEURISY.

When is Aconite indicated in this disease?

High fever, restlessness, sharp stitches in side; chills, especially if brought on by checked perspiration.

In Pleurisy what would be the indications for Bryonia?

Sharp stitching pains in the chest; worse from the slightest motion; friction sounds; lies on affected side.

Mention some other remedies with stitching pains in the chest.

Ranunculus bulb., *Kali carb.*, *Rumex* and *Senega.*

When is Sulphur the remedy?

Sharp stitching pain through left lung; worse lying on back and worse from motion; where well-marked pleuritic effusions refuse to absorb.

Mention another remedy useful to cause absorption of pleuritic fluid.

Apis.

PLEURODYNIA.

What is the chief remedy in this affection, and what are its symptoms?

Ranunculus bulb. There are sharp, sticking pains in

the chest, and a sore spot, worse from motion, pressure or change of temperature.

Where the bruised, sore feeling of the chest walls predominate, what is the remedy?

Arnica.

What are some other drugs sometimes called for in this affection?

Gaultheria, Actæa rac., Rhus rad., Senega and *Rumex.*

When is Bryonia the remedy?

When there is a rheumatic diathesis with stitching, tearing pains; worse by motion; relieved by lying on painful side.

PNEUMONIA.

When is Aconite indicated in Pneumonia?

Where there is high fever preceded by a chill with full, hard and tense pulse, and a hard, dry, teasing and painful cough.

Is there any expectoration under Aconite; if so, what is it?

It is only a serous, frothy or watery expectoration, never thick, but it may be blood tinged.

When does Aconite cease to be useful?

When exudation is commencing, as indicated by thick expectoration.

What other indications do we find under Aconite?

There is great restlessness, tossing about, anxiety, and perhaps fear of death.

How is Aconite distinguished from Veratrum viride?

In commencing pneumonia. Under *Veratrum* we have a full, rapid pulse, indicating great arterial excitement. The eyes are glistening, and there is a red streak along the centre of the tongue.

What is a still further indication of Aconite in Pneumonia?

Especially if it be sudden in its onset and occurs in young, plethoric persons, who are full of life and vigor.

When is Ferrum phos. indicated in first stage of Pneumonia?

When there is a high fever on the onset of the disease, hurried breathing and thin, watery and blood streaked expectoration, and it is useful when the second stage has commenced.

How do we distinguish Ferrum phos. from Aconite?

There is less restlessness and anxiety than under *Aconite*.

Another remedy for first stage is Iodine, what are its symptoms?

It has high fever and restlessness like *Aconite*. There is a tendency to a rapid extension of the hepatization. There is cough and difficulty in breathing as if the chest would not expand, and the sputum is blood streaked.

What are the symptoms of Sanguinaria?

There is a great deal of fever, burning and fullness in the chest. A dry cough, sharp, sticking pains and rust-colored expectoration. There is great arterial excitement also with this drug.

How does it differ here from Veratrum viride?

Under *Veratrum viride* there is little or no hepatization, while *Sanguinaria* is the remedy for hepatization.

What other drug has rust-colored expectoration?

Phosphorus.

What are the symptoms of Sanguinaria in imperfect resolution after Pneumonia?

There is purulent expectoration and it is very offensive, even becoming so to the patient himself.

When does Bryonia come in in Pneumonia?

After *Aconite*, *Ferrum phos.* and *Verat. viride.*

When does Bryonia come in after Aconite?

Bryonia comes in after *Aconite* when the skin is not so hot, nor the face so red, nor the patient so restless, and the cough is not so dry and teasing; then, too, with *Aconite* we have the anxious expression of pulmonary congestion.

What are some other symptoms of Bryonia in Pneumonia?

There are the sharp, stitching, pleuritic pains. There is the hard and dry cough and scanty expectoration, and the patient desires to keep perfectly still, and it is perhaps more indicative in the croupous form of pneumonia. The patient dreads to cough and holds his breath on account of the pain it causes. The patient is relieved by lying on the painful side, because it relieves the motion. Another indication for *Bryonia* is where the cough hurts different parts of the body; for instance, the head.

What are the indications for Kali muriaticum in Pneumonia?

They are mostly clinical. It is given simply on account of the pathological condition, being a fibrinous exudation into the lung substance. The expectoration is white and viscid.

What are the characteristics of Phosphorus in Pneumonia?

It is the remedy when the bronchial symptoms are prominent. There is a cough and a characteristic pressure across the upper part of the chest. There is labored respiration, rust-colored sputum, and it is especially the remedy if typhoid symptoms be present. There is a sensation as if the chest were full of blood, which causes oppression of breathing.

How does the chest oppression of Phosphorus differ from that of Sulphur?

In *Phosphorus* it is external, as of a load *on* the chest. In *Sulphur* it is internal, as if congestion *in* the chest with dyspnœa and burning.

Mention another drug that has weight on the chest but where there is little inflammation.

Ferrum met.

What are the indications for Kali carb. in Pneumonia?

There are sharp, stitching pains in the chest, intense dyspnœa and a great deal of mucus in chest, which is raised with difficulty. The cough is tormenting and there is a great deal of wheezing and whistling breathing.

How do the stitching pains of Bryonia compare with those of Kali carb.?

Like *Bryonia*, they are worse from motion, but unlike *Bryonia* they come whether the patient moves or not, and are more about the lower part of the lung.

When does Kali carb. come in in expectoration?

It comes in after *Ipecac* and *Antimonium tartaricum* have failed to cause the expectoration to be raised.

Give the indications for Chelidonium in Pneumonia.

Here we have stitching pains, especially under the right scapula; the cough is loose and rattling; there is difficult expectoration and oppression in the chest. It is especially the remedy in catarrhal pneumonia of young children where there is plentiful secretion and inability to raise it; it is also the great remedy in bilious pneumonia. The respiration is difficult and there is a fan-like motion of the wings of the nose.

What other drug has the latter symptom, and is it ever indicative in Pneumonia?

Lycopodium. It is a remedy in typhoid pneumonia and for maltreated pneumonia, especially if there be impending suppuration of the lungs. The fan-like motion of the alae nasi the indicative symptom of the drug.

How does Mercurius compare with Chelidonium in bilious Pneumonia?

They are very similar; the stools will decide; the *Mercurius* stool is slimy and attended with tenesmus, occurring both before, during and after stool; the *Mercurius* expectoration is blood streaked, and there are sharp pains from the lower part of the right lung; icteroid symptoms are present.

Give the indications for Antimonium tartaricum.

It is especially indicated in the stage of resolution; there are fine, moist râles heard all over the hepatized portion of the lungs, and there is great oppression of breathing, worse toward morning, compelling the patient to sit up; there is a characterizing symptom in that the patient thinks the next cough will raise the mucus, but it does not do it. There is a great deal of rattling on the chest also.

How does Ipecac differ from Antimonium tart.?

Under *Ipecac* the râles are coarse and large, instead of small and fine, and with *Ipecac* there is always nausea.

When should Sulphur be given in Pneumonia?

Sulphur should be given when the case has a typhoid tendency, and the lung tends to break down; where there are râles, and muco-purulent expectoration, dry tongue and symptoms of hectic fever; there is no tendency to recuperation.

When would Lachesis be indicated in Pneumonia?

Especially when it assumes a typhoid form and where an abscess forms on the lung; brain symptoms are present, such as low muttering, delirium, hallucinations; the sputum is frothy and mixed with blood; the patient rouses out of a sleep in an asthmatic paroxysm.

Is Digitalis ever a remedy for Pneumonia?

Pneumonias in old people with a prune-juice expectoration, cold extremities; cyanotic face and feeble pulse will indicate it. Dyspnœa, the least movement causes palpitation.

When is Hepar indicated?

Late in the disease, when during resolution pus forms; croupous pneumonia.

PREGNANCY, DISORDERS OF.

Mention the principal symptoms of Pulsatilla in the pregnant state.

Threatened abortion, changeable character of the labor

pains; faintness and oppression of the chest; retained placenta from too weak contraction of the uterus.

What is the principal sphere of action of Actea and what are the characteristic symptoms here?

The female sexual organs, and especially in the pregnant state. The symptoms are pain going across the abdomen from hip to hip, seeming to double the patient up. Spasmodic after-pains, and a predisposition to abortion, with nervousness, weeping mood. Ovarian neuralgia, with other reflex, left-sided pains.

What are the symptoms of Bryonia in the pregnant state?

Suppressed lochia, with the splitting headache characteristic of the drug.

What of its use in Milk Fever?

The breasts are hard and tender; there is chilliness, headache, fever, coated tongue, bitter taste and aching in the back and limbs.

What are the indications for Pulsatilla in Milk Fever?

Breasts swollen and painful, with scanty, almost suppressed flow of milk to them, and accompanied by the gloomy, tearful disposition.

Give some indications for the use of Cerium oxalate.

Vomiting of pregnancy or vomiting that is reflex from intestinal or cerebral irritation, spasmodic in character.

What are some uses for Aconite here?

Milk fever; mammary glands hot and swollen; skin hot and dry; suppression of lochia when caused by some violent emotion.

What are the symptoms calling for Caulophyllum?

False labor pains during the latter months of pregnancy; painful bearing-down sensations in hypogastrium.

For what may Hamamelis be used?

For varicose veins over the abdomen, with soreness; and for *phlegmasia alba dolens* or milk leg.

Mention another remedy useful for varices of the pregnant state.

Lycopodium.

What is a useful remedy for toothache of pregnant women?

Magnesia carb.

What are the indications for Nux vomica in morning sickness?

The retching predominates over vomiting. Jaundice may be present, at least the skin is sallow, the bowels are constipated and the appetite lost.

PUERPERAL STATE.

When is Aconite the remedy in Puerperal Fever?

When chill, fever, distended abdomen, suppressed milk, etc., result from too cold bathing or carelessness in changing clothes immediately after delivery.

What are the indications for Actea racemosa in Puerperal Mania?

Patient thinks she will go crazy, is suspicious, has visions of rats, of which she is conscious, but is unable to prevent them.

What are the symptoms of Belladonna in the puerperal state?

Puerperal metritis, with cerebral irritation. Pungent heat of body, abdomen hot, lochia scanty or suppressed. Least jar aggravates. Puerperal eclampsia.

Give symptoms of Gelsemium in impending puerperal convulsions.

There is drowsiness and twitching of different parts of the body, with rigid os. Albuminuria may be present.

How does Veratrum viride compare?

Here the face is red, the eyes injected and the convulsive twitching is more violent.

When is Glonoine the remedy?

In the congestive form of convulsions during labor; where there is much rush of blood to the head, the face is bright red and puffed; patient froths at the mouth and is unconscious.

Name some other remedies sometimes indicated by their general symptoms in Puerperal Convulsions.

Hyoscyamus, Cicuta, Kali brom.

What is a remedy for Puerperal Fever caused by fright?

Opium.

RHEUMATISM.

Give the rheumatic symptoms of Rhus tox.

All *Rhus tox.* rheumatic symptoms are relieved by motion, worse from sitting and worse from rising from a sitting position or first commencing to move; but continued motion relieves, also warmth. They are aggravated during damp weather and are caused by dwelling in damp places. There is stiffness of the muscles and soreness. Prominent projections of the body are sore to touch. It seems to have a special affinity for the deep muscles of the back. It is a remedy also for the effects of over-exertion, such as sprains, wrenches, etc.

What forms of Rheumatism is Ferrum phosphoricum suitable to?

Articular rheumatism or sub-acute rheumatism, the pains are worse from motion.

What drugs have relief from slow motion?

Lycopodium, Pulsatilla and *Ferrum.*

What are the indications for Rhododendron in Rheumatism?

There is great susceptibility to change of weather, particularly changes to cold winter weather. The pains are worse during rest. There is a weak paralytic feeling, and it is especially useful in chronic rheumatism affecting the smaller joints. It is a very useful remedy for rheumatic gout.

Give the symptoms of Ledum in rheumatic troubles.

Pains of *Ledum* characteristically travel upward. It is a remedy for gout and rheumatism affecting the smaller joints. The pains are worse from the warmth of the bed.

How does Ledum compare with Bryonia?

Ledum produces a scanty effusion which tends to harden into nodosities, while *Bryonia* tends to a copious effusion.

What other drugs have nodular swellings in the joints?

Calcarea carb., Benzoic acid, Lycopodium, Ammonium phos. and *Lithium carb.*

What are the rheumatic symptoms of Bryonia?

It is a remedy for acute articular rheumatism with violent local inflammation; the parts being hot, shining and dark or pale red, and the pains are greatly aggravated from motion; external heat relieves.

Give the principal difference between Rhus tox. and Bryonia in rheumatic troubles.

Bryonia is aggravated by motion and *Rhus tox.* is relieved by motion.

Give the rneumatic symptoms of Actea spicata.

It has an affinity for the smaller joints. The joints ache and swell while the patient is walking. It is especially indicated in the rheumatism of hands and feet.

How does this compare with Actea racemosa?

Actea racemosa affects the bellies of the muscles rather than the joints.

What other drug is especially useful for rheumatism of the smaller joints of the hands and feet?

Caulophyllum.

Give the symptoms of Colchicum in rheumatic troubles.

The pains are worse in evening. The affected parts are swollen and dark red, and there is a tendency for the disease to shift about from one joint to another. It is especially useful for rheumatic affections in debilitated persons; those who are weak—weakness being the characteristic.

Give the rheumatic symptoms of Guaiacum.

Chronic forms of rheumatism where the joints become distorted by concretions; contractions of tendons; worse from motion.

What drug has special action on the right wrist?

Viola odorata.

What are the rheumatic symptoms of Kalmia?

Rheumatism affecting the chest and rheumatism which shifts from the joints to the head, especially after external applications to the joints, and the rheumatism of *Kalmia*, unlike that of *Ledum*, travels downwards; useful in heart affections, such as pericarditis and endocarditis from rheumatism.

What are the rheumatic symptoms of Pulsatilla?

The chief characteristic is the wandering of the pains; the disease shifts about from one joint to another; they are worse from warmth and in the evening, and are relieved from cold; the pains are so severe as to compel the patient to move. Rheumatism following an attack of indigestion.

What other drugs have Rheumatism which shifts about?

Kali sulph., *Kali bich.*, *Sulphur*, *Bryonia*, *Colchicum* and *Kalmia*.

What are the rheumatic pains of Ranunculus bulbosus?

The pains are worse in damp weather, and particularly from a change of weather and change of temperature; intercostal rheumatism, stitch in side and a feeling as if parts were pounded.

Give the rheumatic symptoms of Causticum.

Causticum is useful where the joints are stiff and where the tendons are shortened; rheumatoid arthritis calls for the drug, and the pains of *Causticum* are worse from cold and relieved from warmth; restlessness at night; drawing muscular pains; the parts on which he lies become sore.

How can we distinguish Rhus tox from Causticum?

Rhus tox. has restlessness and relief from motion all the time; with *Causticum* there is only nocturnal restlessness.

What drug has rheumatic pains which make the patients almost beside themselves, compelling them to get out of bed and walk about?

Chamomilla.

Three other drugs, Rhus tox., Ferrum met. and Veratrum alb., have rheumatic pains relieved by moving about; how are they distinguished from Chamomilla?

They all lack the feverishness, excitement and irritability of *Chamomilla*.

What are the rheumatic indications for Dulcamara?

It is useful in rheumatism made worse from change of weather. That is the chief characteristic of the drug. Rheumatic pains of the muscles from taking cold during the prevalence of damp, raw weather.

What are the indications for Sulphur in Rheumatism?

It is indicated in acute and chronic rheumatism when the inflammatory swellings seem to ascend—that is, they commence in the feet and extend up the body; the pains are worse in bed and at night, and it is especially a remedy for jerking of the limbs in falling off to sleep during a course of acute rheumatism.

What are the symptoms of Benzoic acid in Rheumatism?

It is a remedy for rheumatism and gout with extremely offensive urine, and especially is it useful for rheumatism of the smaller joints; gouty nodosities, weeping sinews.

When is Kali hydriodicum indicated in Rheumatism?

When the pains are worse at night when lying on affected side, and when the troubles are of mercurial or specific origin.

What are the indications for Silicea in Rheumatism?

It is one of the best remedies in chronic hereditary rheumatism. The pains are worse at night and worse from uncovering; better from warmth.

What are the rheumatic symptoms of Sanguinaria?

Sanguinaria gives a picture of acute muscular rheumatism ; the pains are shifting, sharp and stitching, with great soreness and stiffness in the muscles, especially those of the back and neck ; rheumatism of right deltoid muscle.

What remedies have special affinity for the left deltoid muscle?

Ferrum metallicum and *Nux moschata*.

What other drug is useful for Rheumatism of the right shoulder, also with rheumatic pains which are worse after a long walk ; better from warmth, but worse in bed?

Magnesia carb.

What are the symptoms calling for Apis mel.?

The affected parts feel very stiff and sore to pressure, and there is a sensation of numbness ; the joints affected are swollen, and there is a sensation as if the skin over them were stretched tight: the swelling is apt to be rather pale than red, and there is usually a great deal of effusion into the joints. It is especially a remedy for synovitis.

Give the symptoms of Belladonna in Rheumatism.

There are cutting lightning-like pains running along the joints; the joints are swollen, red and shining, and pain radiates through the inflamed joints. It is one of the best remedies in rheumatic stiffness caused by getting the head and neck wet or sitting with the head and neck exposed to a draft.

What are the rheumatic symptoms indicating Calcarea carb?

It is useful for rheumatic affections caused by working in the water and for rheumatism of the muscles of the back and shoulders after *Rhus tox.* fails.

Give indications for Ruta graveolens in Rheumatism.

Soreness and lameness as from a sprain or bruise. Rheumatism of wrists and ankles.

Mention some drugs having a weakness or giving away of the ankles.

Causticum, *Sulphuric acid*, *Sulphur* and *Silicea*.

What remedy is especially indicated in Rheumatism of the fleshy parts of the muscles?

Actea racemosa.

What are the rheumatic symptoms of Arnica?

Rheumatism resulting from exposure to dampness, cold and excessive muscular strain combined; the parts are sore and bruised.

SCARLET FEVER.

When is Ailanthus indicated in Scarlet fever?

When the patient lies in a stupor; rash is imperfect, dark and purplish; swollen throat and infiltration of the cellular tissue about the neck; excoriating nasal discharge; drowsiness and prostration; thin, bloody, offensive stools.

What indicates Belladonna in Scarlet fever?

Smooth, bright red rash, the cerebral irritation, the sore throat, the strawberry tongue and the swelling of the glands.

What of the prophylactic power of Belladonna?

Hahnemann discovered that Belladonna was a prophylactic in scarlet fever, and it has certainly been verified clinically.

When should Bryonia be given?

When the rash suddenly disappears and alarming symptoms occur such as a typhoid tendency. Also when the rash appears slowly.

When should Rhus be given in Scarlet fever?

When the child is drowsy, restless, has a red and smooth tongue, œdematous fauces and enlarged glands; eruption does not come out and is miliary; great depression and weakness,

How does Ailanthus compare here?

The rash is dark-bluish, the throat is swollen, there is an acrid nasal discharge and the child is drowsy and stupid.

When is Zincum indicated in Scarlatina and other eruptive diseases?

When the patient is very weak, too weak in fact to develop an eruption, and as a result there are often brain symptoms, such as meningitis, with sharp pains through the head.

Give symptoms of Lachesis in Scarlet fever.

When the rash is slowly and imperfectly developed, dark and accompanied with diphtheritic deposits; pulse weak, surface dark, and perhaps hemorrhages.

Give indications for Apis in Scarlatina.

The fever is high, no thirst, blisters on border of tongue; patient is puffy and drowsy; urine scanty; skin prickly; restlessness and nervous agitation.

What are the symptoms calling for Muriatic acid?

In malignant cases with ulceration of the throat, acrid discharges from the nose, eruption faint and livid, flushed cheeks, fetid breath.

SCIATICA.

Give symptoms of Colocynth in Sciatica.

Sharp, spasmodic attacks of pain shoot down the sciatic nerve to the feet; crampy pains as if the parts were screwed in a vise; it is worse on the right side and at night, and tends to be paroxysmal; relieved by warmth and rest; aggravated by motion. The nerves around the hip joint and acetabulum suffer most severely.

How does Gnaphalium compare here?

Intense pains along sciatic nerve, with numbness, which sometimes alternates with the pains; pains extend to toes. Rheumatic pains in toes. Better sitting in chair.

Give briefly characteristic indications for Kali bich., Kali hyd. and Phytolacca in Sciatica.

Kali bich. Darting pains in left side; *relieved by motion.*
Kali hyd. Pains worse at night from lying on affected

side, and especially when of mercurial or syphilitic origin.

Phytolacca. Pains darting and tearing; *aggravated by motion.*

What drug has Sciatic pains worse while sitting, somewhat relieved by walking, and entirely relieved by lying down?

Ammonium mur.

When is Rhus the remedy?

In chronic cases brought on by exposure to wet; straining and lifting pains worse at rest, relieved by motion, heat and rubbing.

Give indications for Cimicifuga in this affection.

Lancing pains in left hip. Pains become so acute as to drive patient out of bed; better sitting, relieved by pressure.

SCROFULA.

What are the symptoms of Iodine in Scrofulosis?

Where there is great induration of the glands, they are very sluggish and torpid; the patient is subject to wasting diseases, there is wasting of the mammæ, ovaries. testicles, etc.

Give some indications for Sulphur in Scrofula.

Tendency to eruptions; defective osseous growth; open fontanelles; bone affections; rickets and curvature of the spine. Appetite voracious, caused by defective assimilation from diseased glands. The child looks like a little old man or woman; the skin is wrinkled and flabby.

When is Graphites the remedy?

When the lymphatic glands of the neck and axillæ are swollen; also the inguinal and mesenteric glands, and when there are marked skin symptoms.

What are the indications for Mercurius in Scrofula?

Enlarged glands; open fontanelles, especially the posterior; slow in learning to walk; imperfect formation of teeth; feet cold and damp; perspiration about head offensive and oily.

Differentiate between Calcarea carb. and Silicea in scrofulous diseases.

The *Calcarea* sweat is mostly about the head and is offensive.

The *Silicea* sweat is especially about the feet and is offensive.

Calcarea is not as sensitive as *Silicea*.

Give some other symptoms of Calcarea.

Dentition is slow. The abdomen is swollen, child is "pot-bellied." The upper lip is swollen. The fontanelles are open. There is emaciation. The skin is flabby and hangs in folds. Partial sweating is characteristic. Scrofulous affections of the bones.

SEASICKNESS.

When should Petroleum be given in Seasickness?

Nausea, which is worse from motion or riding, and accompanied by vertigo; the vertigo comes on especially when the patient raises his eyes; there is also bilious vomiting.

Mention a remedy that clinically has been found useful in Seasickness.

Apomorphia.

Mention a remedy having nausea from any swinging motion or riding in a carriage or the cars.

Cocculus.

SKIN, DISEASES OF.

What are the skin symptoms of Rhus tox.?

The skin is red and covered with numerous vesicles. There is great itching and tingling. The skin is swollen and œdematous. It is especially the remedy for vesicular erysipelas.

How does Apis differ from Rhus tox.?

Under *Apis* there is more burning and stinging than under *Rhus.* There is also more œdema, and in erysipelas it is more especially indicated in the pale variety than in the vesicular variety.

What are the symptoms of Cantharis in skin troubles?

Cantharis produces large blisters on the skin, and there is especially a great deal of burning and smarting. The blisters are the characteristic. Burns and scalds.

What is the eruption of Croton tiglium?

The blisters are very small and numerous and itch terribly, and they form pustules which dry into yellow scabs, the characteristics being the confluent vesicles and the itching accompanying.

What is a similar remedy here?

Hura Brasiliensis.

What are the symptoms of Ranunculus bulbosus?

It forms vesicles of the skin, which are filled with serum and burn. They sometimes have a bluish-black appearance, and it is especially indicated when these vesicles form along the course of the nerves, producing a disease known as shingles. Herpes zoster.

Give the characteristic action of Mezereum.

There are numerous small vesicles with terrible itching, but the characteristic is that the secretion dries quickly, producing thick, high scabs, from which an acrid, thick pus oozes. Crusts and itching are characteristic.

What sort of an eruption does Chininum sulph. cause?

It is called erythematous, and resembles greatly scarlet fever.

Mention another remedy which resembles Cantharis in producing large blisters which burst and leave a raw surface.

Ranunculus sceleratus.

What sort of an eruption is characteristic of the Potashes?

Papulous eruption.

What are the characteristic skin symptoms of Psorinum?

Herpetic eruptions on the skin, accompanied by a great deal of itching, which is worse as soon as patient gets in bed. The skin is dirty, greasy, and looks as if it had never been washed. Tinea capitis; oozing of offensive matter.

What are the chief skin symptoms of Sulphur?

The troubles of the skin are apt to alternate with some internal trouble; there is the great aggravation from washing, and the more the eruption is scratched the more it itches and burns; the skin is rough, coarse and measley; the eruptions are usually pustular, and there is tendency to soreness in the folds of the skin.

Give the scalp symptoms of Sulphur.

Great dryness and heat of the scalp, with intense itching, and scratching, though it relieves, causes burning; all the eruptions are greatly aggravated by washing and by being wet; wetting produces burning; there may be also an eruption of yellow crusts on the scalp.

What are the skin symptoms of Graphites?

Moist, scabby eruptions, especially of the scalp, face, bends of joints, and in the folds of skin, as between the fingers, behind the ears, in the corners of the mouth or eyes; they are cracked, bleeding, or oozing a gluey, honey like, thick and tenacious discharge; the skin may be dry and horny; there is absence of sweat, the hair is dry and falls out, the nails become loose. Cicatrices are benefited by *Graphites*.

What drug has dry, scaly eruptions?

Lycopodium.

What drug has thick, hard, scabby and crusty eruptions?

Mezereum.

What symptoms does Arsenicum produce upon the Skin?

1. Pains, itching, biting, gnawing and burning.
2. Watery swellings, from puffiness to œdema.

3. Eruptions, papules, nettle rash and pimples.

4. Painful ulcers, burning and sensitive, with offensive discharges.

What is the eruption of Oleander?

The skin is sensitive; slight friction causes chafing and soreness. It produces eruption on the scalp and back of the ears like a crusta lactea, which oozes a fluid and breeds vermin.

How does Vinca minor compare here?

This also produces an eruption which breeds vermin and it produces by the discharge a matted condition of the hair, and there is a very offensive odor arising therefrom. Eczema of scalp and face. Plica polonica.

How does Viola tricolor compare?

It is useful for crusts on the scalp where the exudation is very copious. It mats the hair like *Vinca minor* and is distinguished by its urinary symptoms; urine smells like that of a cat.

What is the characteristic of the Staphisagria eruption?

It is worse on the occiput, and the characteristic indication is that it itches terribly, but scratching changes the place of the itching.

What two other drugs have this last symptom, though less marked?

Anacardium and *Mezereum*.

Mention two other drugs useful for Crusta lactea.

Nux juglans and *Arctium lappa*.

What are the skin symptoms of Petroleum?

Petroleum has an eruption which particularly occurs behind the ears; it is a pure eczema; the skin is harsh and dry, and there are deep cracks and fissures which bleed and suppurate; the finger tips are cracked and painful and the hands chap.

How is Petroleum distinguished from Graphites in its Skin symptoms?

Graphites pictures more of a herpes and *Petroleum* more of an eczema.

What are the skin symptoms of Natrum muriaticum?

It is a dry, scaly eruption, or a herpetic eruption of little watery blisters; especially when in the bends of the knees; also, it is a remedy for affections of the scalp accompanied by a falling of the hair and the brows. Eruptions on flexor surfaces.

What drug has eruptions on the extensor surfaces?

Kreasote.

What are the indications for Apis in Urticaria?

The eruption suddenly appears on the surface of the skin in long pinkish-white welts, with terrible itching.

What two drugs are especially useful for Urticaria caused by eating shell fish?

Urtica urens and *Terebinth.*

What is the action of Sepia on the Skin?

It causes yellowish-brown spots on the skin with itching, redness and rawness. It is especially a remedy for ringworms. Herpetic conditions about knees and ankles.

Mention two other drugs useful for Ringworms.

Tellurium and *Calcarea carb.*

What are the indications for Belladonna in skin diseases?

It causes a bright scarlet redness of the skin, which is

extremely sensitive to the touch. It has an erysipelatous condition, and there is a great deal of throbbing, as if the deeper parts of the skin were affected.

What is the action of Anacardium on the Skin?

It is useful where the skin is covered with small blisters, which have an umbilicated center; they discharge a yellow serum which hardens into crusts with extreme itchiness. It is one of the antidotes to *Rhus* poisoning.

Mention three other drugs useful for Rhus poisoning.

Croton tiglium, *Ammonium carb.* and *Grindelia robusta*.

What of Anacardium occidentale or the Cashew nut?

Useful in a vesicular eruption on the skin, which is umbilicated and which itches terribly.

Give the skin symptoms of Antimonium crudum.

It produces thick, horny collosities on the skin; it causes deficient growth of the nails, and the eruptions are crusty—the crusts being of a honey yellow character; the skin cracks easily.

Give a remedy which produces Acne.

Kali bromatum.

What are three remedies for Psoriasis?

Arsenic, *Arsenicum iodide* and *Rhus tox*.

Mention a use of Thuja in skin affections.

It is a remedy for warts and diseases of the epidermal tissue, such as affections of the nails, etc.

How do the Warts calling for Thuja differ from those calling for Causticum?

The *Causticum* warts have a solid body and are very

horny. *Thuja* warts are fissured, cut up, having a cauliflower appearance.

What is the action of Arnica on the Skin?

It produces a peculiar form of erysipelas—a dermatitis with much itching and soreness, dark blue in color. Boils with great soreness.

What remedy antidotes the skin symptoms of Arnica?

Camphor.

Why should Arnica be diluted before being applied externally?

Because the tincture is resinous and not only liable to produce the condition above referred to in sensitive skins, but this quality interferes with its easy absorption.

What action has Calcarea upon the Skin?

The skin is unhealthy; small wounds suppurate easily; it is useful for certain forms of eczema of the scalp with general *Calcarea* symptoms.

What is our principal use of Comocladia dentata?

It has many symptoms on the skin similar to *Rhus tox.*, but its peculiar symptom is a pain in the right eye as if it were pushed out of the head; worse near a warm stove.

What is our use of Dolichos, another of the same family?

A violent itching all over the body without any visible eruption; useful in intense itching of jaundice, which is worse at night.

What effect has Dulcamara on the Skin?

It produces an eruption of large wheals, and it is useful in such be brought on by digestive troubles, with aggravation from cold air.

What are the skin symptoms of Hepar?

The skin is sensitive to the open air; inflamed skin; injuries suppurate easily; eruptions and ulcerations are sensitive, and bleed easily, and discharge a foul smelling excretion; around the principal ulcerations there are little pimples.

What symptoms has Hippomane mancinella?

It produces vesicles on the skin, with an intense erythema; so irritating is it that water dropping from its leaves on the skin will produce vesicles. It has been utilized in scarlet fever when this intense irritation of the skin exists.

What is Hydrocotyle Asiatica used for?

Skin diseases, with an immense amount of desquammation.

Tell the uses of Sarsaparilla.

Sycotic eruptions looking like the roseola of syphilis and itching intolerably; eruptions exuding an irritating pus; moist eruption about genitals. Is an anti-sycotic remedy.

What, in general, are the skin symptoms of Silicea?

There is a general unhealthy condition of the skin. It suppurates easily and heals with difficulty. In suppurative skin diseases it is our best remedy.

What is the action of Tartar emetic on the Skin?

It produces an eruption of pustules resembling those of smallpox, for which it is a remedy.

What are the indications for Urtica urens?

Nettle rash, with intolerable itching and burning;

hives from eating shell fish. Also indicated in absence of milk after confinement without apparent cause.

What are the indications for Viola tricolor in Eczema?

Crusta lactea, with copious exudation which mats the hair, and urine smelling like that of a cat.

Mention two remedies for Eczema of the dorsa of the hands.

Natrum carb. and *Pix liquida.*

SLEEPLESSNESS.

Give indications for Ambra in sleeplessness.

Sleeplessness due to worry about business matters, with spasms and twitching of the muscles, especially in thin, spare, nervous men.

Give the indications for Chamomilla in the sleeplessness of children.

They start during sleep, the muscles of the hands and face twitch; there may be colic; and the face, especially one cheek, is red.

What should be given if in addition there is delirium?

Belladonna.

When is Ignatia called for in Insomnia?

Where hyperæmia of the brain is brought on by depressing emotion such as grip.

Give symptoms of Cypripedium in sleeplessness.

Children awake at night and are lively and full of play. It indicates impending cerebral trouble.

What is the sleeplessness calling for Coffea?

It is where the patient is quiet and sleepless, where the

senses are all acute, hears distant noises with great distinctness, the mind is active with plans and fancies, and the next day the patient is tremulous; also where hyperæsthesia of the skin keeps him awake.

What action has Ferrum phosphoricum on sleep?

In low potencies it has been found to cause sleeplessness, and in higher potencies it has been used with success in sleeplessness, especially when caused by a hyperæmic condition of the brain.

Give the indications of Hyoscyamus in sleeplessness in children.

They twitch and scream out in the sleep as if frightened, the brain is full of bewildering images.

Give the sleep symptoms of Nux.

Sleepy in the evening, falls asleep in his chair, and falls asleep immediately on going to bed; wakes an hour or so before daybreak; dozes off again and awakes more tired than he was before going to bed, and with a headache. Insomnia from abuse of stimulants.

How does Pulsatilla compare?

The *Pulsatilla* patient is wide awake in the evening, but the sleep is sound and the patient awakes languid, or else there is restless sleep with troubled dreams.

What is characteristic about the sleep of Sulphur?

The patient sleeps in "cat naps;" the slightest noise awakens, and there is great difficulty in falling asleep again.

What is the sleeplessness of Cocculus?

From pure mental activity slight loss of sleep causes sickness.

What is the sleeplessness of Gelsemium?

Patients are dull and stupid, seem on the verge of slumber, but unable to sleep. Nervous system exhausted.

SORE THROAT.

What are the throat symptoms of Ammonium causticum?

Aphonia, with burning rawness in the throat.

What are the indications for Baptisia in Sore Throat?

Solids cause gagging; excessive putridity, ulcerations with an excessively offensive odor from the mouth and throat.

What are the indications for Belladonna in Sore Throat?

Great dryness and bright redness of the throat, the fauces are inflamed, the tonsils are swollen and enlarged, worse on the right side; food and liquids are ejected through the nose on swallowing.

What are the indications for Capsicum in Sore Throat?

Sore throat of smokers and drinkers with burning and relaxed uvula, throat sore and contracted even when not swallowing.

What are the throat symptoms of Cantharis?

Burning from the mouth to the stomach; throat highly inflamed and covered with plastic lymph; spasm of the throat and intense constriction about the throat.

When should Cistus Canadensis be thought of in throat troubles?

The keynote is intense dryness, the patient has to get up at night to drink to allay this dryness. There is a sensation of sand in the throat, and submaxillary glands are swollen.

Give the throat symptoms of Ferrum phosphoricum.

Dry, red, inflamed and painful throat; sore throat of singers and speakers.

What are the throat symptoms of Gelsemium?

Aphonia from paresis of the muscles, sore scraped throat accompanying nasal symptoms; pain extends into ears, worse right side; postdiphtheritic paralysis.

Give indications for Guaiacum in Sore Throat.

Worse on right side; swollen tonsils; enlarged veins; must drink to assist deglutition, as throat is dry; stinging pains in throat, worse in warm, moist air.

What are the throat symptoms of Hepar?

Sharp splinter-like pains in the throat, or a sensation as if there were a lump in the throat. Tonsillitis with tendency to suppuration.

What other drugs have sticking pains in the throat?

Argentum nitricum and *Nitric acid*.

What are the throat symptoms of Ignatia?

There is a lump in the throat and a sticking sensation, which is relieved by swallowing.

Give indications for Kali bichromicum in the throat.

There is a great swelling of the tonsils and ulcers which secrete a purulent discharge; there are diseased follicles which exude a caseous matter; the coating of the tongue is yellow at the base; the discharge is ropy, tenacious and stringy.

When is Kali muriaticum indicated in Sore Throat?

Follicular pharyngitis with gray or white exudation; tonsils swollen and inflamed, grayish spots, patches or ulcers in the throat; ulcerated sore throat; swelling of the glands about the throat. It has proved a very useful remedy in diphtheria.

Give the characteristic throat symptoms of Lachesis.

Sensation of lump in left side of the throat, which seems to go down when swallowing, but returns again; constriction of throat and difficult breathing, worse on arousing from sleep or after sleep; empty swallowing is painful and fluids escape from the nose; throat sensitive externally.

What are the indications for Lycopodium in throat troubles?

Enlarged tonsils, which are studded with small ulcers. It holds the same relation to the right side of the throat that *Lachesis* does to the left; diphtheritic deposits on the right side of the throat; tonsils and tongue are both swollen.

Give the characteristics of Mercurius in Sore Throat.

Dryness and great soreness in the throat; the patient is obliged to swallow constantly, and there is great soreness and swelling of the glands externally.

What are the indications for Mercurius proto-iodide in throat affections?

Diphtheritic deposits beginning on the right side, with great swelling of the glands, and accumulation of thick, tenacious mucus in the throat; the tongue is coated yellow at the base, the tip and sides being red.

Give indications for Mercurius biniodide in throat affections.

Sore throat, just like the *Proto-iodide*, except that it is worse on the left side; there is more glandular swelling and more fever than in the *Proto-iodide*, thus partaking more of the features of *Iodine*.

What are the throat symptoms of Mercurius corrosivus?

The uvula is swollen, and there is intense burning, worse from pressure; constriction of the throat, swallowing causes spasm.

What condition of the throat calls for Natrum mur.?

A relaxed uvula with a feeling of a plug or great dryness in the throat.

What throat affections correspond to Nux?

Those of smokers, drinkers and preachers; there is a follicular rawness and scraping from overuse of the voice.

What are the throat symptoms of Nitric acid?

Sensation of a splinter, fishbone or piece of glass in the throat, ulcers in the throat with offensive discharges and odor.

What are the throat symptoms of Phytolacca?

Dry, sore throat of dark red color; the tonsils are dark red; pain on swallowing, especially at the root of the tongue, accompanied by general aching in the back and limbs.

How is the appearance of the throat under Sulphuric acid?

There is a white membrane in the throat, throat looks as if it was whitewashed.

Give symptoms of Alumina in Sore Throat.

Relaxed throat; clergyman's sore throat; dark red throat with elongated uvula; sensation of a splinter in throat when swallowing.

What other drugs have this splinter-like sensation?

Hepar, *Argentum nitr.*, *Nitric acid* and *Carbo veg*.

What is a characteristic throat symptom of all the Potashes?

An accumulation of tough, tenacious mucus in the throat; the patient hems and hawks to clear throat in the morning.

SPERMATORRHŒA.

What is the characteristic use of Agnus castus?

Spermatorrhœa and sexual excesses in "old sinners," with loss of sexual power and coldness of the genital organs.

Give the characteristic indications for Bufo rana, a South American toad, sometimes used in medicine.

For masturbation, where the patient seeks solitude to perform the act; epilepsy caused by sexual intercourse, the aura seeming to start from the sexual organs.

What do we use Caladium for?

Effects of sexual excesses, where there are emissions without any excitement. Penis is flabby, prepuce remains when retracted.

What are the sexual symptoms of Conium?

Enfeebled state of the sexual organs from masturbation, and hypochondriasis therefrom; emissions from the slightest provocation.

Give indications for the use of Eryngium.

Seminal weakness, with discharge of prostatic fluid from slight causes.

What are the male sexual symptoms of Gelsemium?

Prostration and loss of tone in the sexual organs; coldness; spermatorrhœa without erections, impotence, involuntary emissions resulting from masturbation; gonorrhœa in the beginning, with marked soreness at the mouth of the urethra; discharge scanty, little pain, but much heat.

What affection about the sexual sphere corresponds to Lycopodium?

Impotence, with cold, relaxed sexual organs, and diminished sexual power.

When is Nuphar to be thought of?

When there is total impotence, complete loss of sexual desire.

Give indications for Nux in sexual excesses.

Frequent emissions, towards night backache and difficulty of walking.

Give the male sexual symptoms of Phosphorus.

Increased sexual desire, followed by loss of sexual desire and emissions; the patient has desire and fancies, but no power.

What are the male sexual symptoms of Phosphoric acid?

Debility, relaxation or impotence from sexual excesses, frequent weak emissions and dragging pains in the testicles; weakness in back and legs and burning spine; spermatorrhœa.

What are the sexual symptoms of Picric acid?

Excitement, priapism and profuse emissions, erections very violent; legs are heavy; there is prostration from least exertion; erections keep the patient awake at night.

Give the sexual symptoms of Selenium.

Spermatorrhœa, with irritability, mental confusion, headache and paralytic weakness of the spine; the system is so relaxed that the semen dribbles away.

What are the symptoms calling for Zincum?

Spermatorrhœa from long-lasting abuse, with hypochondriasis, pale, sunken countenance, eyes surrounded by blue rings; testicles drawn up.

What are the indications for Calcarea in sexual excesses?

Excessive sexual desire, rather more mental than physical; erections are imperfect, emission is premature; night sweats follow emissions.

How does Sulphur compare?

Patient is debilitated; frequent nocturnal emissions; semen is thin and watery; organs are relaxed, emissions too soon; there is backache, weakness and hypochondriasis.

Give symptoms calling for Lycopodium.

Complete impotence; erections are absent or imperfect; genitals cold and shriveled.

What are the indications for Staphisagria?

Effects of masturbation; dark rings under eyes, sallow face, peevish and shy; depressed mental condition from allowing the mind to dwell too much on sexual subjects.

SPINAL IRRITATION.

What are the indications for Agaricus in Spinal Irritation?

Tingling and formication in the back; itching or biting of the skin as if frost bitten; twitching of muscles and sensation as if needles of ice were thrust into the skin.

When is Chininum sulph. indicated in Spinal Irritation?

Where there is great sensitiveness of the spine in the dorsal region; the last cervical and first dorsal vertebræ are very sensitive to pressure.

Give indications for Zincum in Spinal Irritation.

There is aching about the last dorsal or first lumbar vertebra, worse when sitting; there is burning along the spine and trembling of the limbs.

Give indications for Physostigma.

All the spinal nerves are irritated, pressure between vertebræ, causes patient to wince. There is burning and tingling, and numbness of hands and feet, and jerking of the limbs on falling asleep.

Give indications for Actea rac. in Spinal Irritation.

The cervical vertebræ are sensitive to pressure; patient cannot lean back in chair; the symptoms are usually reflex from uterine troubles.

How does Natrum mur. compare?

Pressure on back, even lying on something hard relieves the patient. Paralysis from weakness of the spine.

What are the indications for Cocculus Indicus?

Paralytic aching in small of back, with an empty gone feeling in stomach.

Give symptoms calling for Phosphorus.

The spine is sensitive; the back and limbs are weak; patient stumbles easily; often these symptoms result from a loss of animal fluids.

SPLEEN, DISEASES OF.

What is the action of Quinine on the Spleen?

It enlarges it, hence may be useful in enlargement of that organ.

What is the action of Ceanothus on the Spleen?

It enlarges it, producing a persistent pain in the left hypochondrium, with intense dyspnœa.

Give symptoms of Grindelia robusta, another spleen remedy.

Sore, aching or cutting pain in region of spleen extending as low down as hip; spleen large and tender; sallow complexion.

Mention three remedies useful for swollen spleen from malarial poison.

Aranea diad., *Cinchona* and *Chininum sulph.*

SUNSTROKE.

Give symptoms of Glonoine in Sunstroke.

Face pale, full, round pulse, labor respiration, eyes fixed, cerebral vomiting, white tongue, sinking at the pit of the stomach.

What are the symptoms calling for Natrum carbonicum in the effects of summer weather?

Debility and headache from the sun; chronic effects of sunstroke; the *Natrum carb.* patient gets very nervous during thunder storms and hides in the cellar; this nervousness is said to be due to the electrical condition of the atmosphere acting on such patients.

Give indications for Lachesis.

Hot weather fatigues. Face is dark red, sunken and cadaverous; extremities are cold; sun makes him languid, dizzy and faint.

SYNOVITIS.

What are the indications for Apis in Synovitis?

Sharp lancinating, stinging pains shooting through the joint; worse from slightest motion and better from cold applications.

How does Bryonia compare?

The pains are more stitching, with tension, and better from warmth. Synovitis caused by cold or an injury.

When is Sulphur indicated?

When there is effusion. It produces absorption.

SYPHILIS.

Give the symptoms calling for the use of Mercurius in Syphilitic affections.

Sore throat of secondary syphilis, soft chancres and buboes. Nocturnal syphilitic pains, which come on and banish sleep as soon as the patient goes to bed.

In what Syphilitic conditions is Mercurius protoiodide useful?

Iritis, and painless hard chancres; with swelling of the inguinal glands.

Give general difference between Hepar and Mercurius.

Both are sensitive to cold air, both sweat easily, both have tendency to suppurations, but only *Mercury* has the nocturnal pains.

Give some indications for Nitric acid in Syphilis.

Secondary syphilis; phagedenic chancres; soreness of the skin and cranial bones, worse from damp weather; ulcers in the throat, irregular in outline; yellowish-brown or copper-colored spots over the body.

What are the chief uses of Stillingia?

Syphilis of the long bones, periostitis and ostitis; pain worse at night and in damp weather.

Give symptoms calling for Carbo animalis.

Coppery red blotches on skin, swollen glands, emaciation; after abuse of *Mercury*, buboes which have been opened too soon, leaving a stony hardness around them.

Give the symptoms of Kali hyd.

Gnawing bone pains, papules, ulcerating and leaving scars, rupia; chancres with hard edges. Tertiary syphilis.

What are the indications for Lachesis?

When the chancre is gangrenous, the ulcers are blue, there are nightly bone pains. The ulcers are very sensitive.

Give the indications for Lycopodium.

Coppery eruption on forehead. Indolent chancres. Ulcers refuse to heal; made worse by dressings. Syphilitic ulcers in right side of throat.

TEETH, AFFECTIONS OF.

When is Coffea applicable in Toothache and when Chamomilla?

The toothache of *Coffea* is relieved permanently by holding cold water in the mouth; that of *Chamomilla* is only temporarily relieved.

Give indications for Mercurius in Toothache.

The teeth feel sore, the roots are inflamed, and often there are abscesses at the roots; there is great nocturnal aggravation; increased salivation and sensation as if the teeth were too long or too loose.

What are the symptoms of the teeth calling for Staphisagria?

The teeth turn black and crumble as soon as they appear, a condition found in sycotic children.

What other drug has a premature decay of teeth; they first become yellow and then dark?

Kreasote.

In what affection of the teeth and gums do we find Silicea indicated?

In abscesses about the roots of the teeth and dental fistulæ.

Mention some remedies useful for abscess at the roots of teeth.

Lachesis, Mercurius, Hepar and *Silicea.*

TETANUS.

Mention some nervous symptoms of Physostigma.

It causes tetanic spasms of involuntary muscles. It causes paralysis and diminished reflex action.

What is the difference between death due to Strychnine poison and death due to poisoning by the Calabar bean?

In *Strychnine* death results from asphyxiation caused by tetanic spasm of the respiratory muscles.
Calabar bean causes death by paralysis.

What are some of the nervous symptoms of Strychnine?

The patient has characteristic irritability from external impressions. The slightest jar or noise sends him into spasms. The patient faints from odors. The patient has tetanic spasms and opisthotonos.

What are some of the nervous symptoms of Phytolacca?

There are convulsive symptoms with stiff limbs, clenched teeth, and opisthotonos.

Mention three other remedies for tetanus.

Curare, *Passiflora* and *Angustura*.

How do the symptoms of Picrotoxine differ from those of Strychnine?

Picrotoxine does not have the irritability and sensitiveness to the touch that *Strychnine* has.

How is Stramonium differentiated from Strychnine?

Both cause tetanic convulsions, which is worse from light and touch, but with *Stramonium* mania is almost always present. With *Strychnine* the mind is clear to the last.

What are some useful remedies in impending Tetanus?

Aconite, fever, tingling and numbness.

Verat. vir. and *Hypericum*, where there is excruciating pain in the wound.

Bell., *Cicuta* and *Silicea* when the suppurating wound suddenly ceases to discharge, and tetanic symptoms appear.

Give some indications for Cicuta.

Sudden rigidity and distortion, followed by prostration; spasm renewed by touch; oppression of breathing; fixed stare to eyes.

When is Hydrocyanic acid the remedy?

The body is stiffened and thrown back; cramp in the nape; breathing in paroxysms; set jaws; frothing at the mouth similar to *Nux vomica*, but the face is flushed.

TONSILLITIS.

When is Mercurius the remedy in Tonsillitis?

When pus is forming, it favors its evacuation and formation, as it does in all conditions of abscess.

When is Silicea indicated in Tonsillitis?

When there is suppuration; when the abscess is broken and the suppurative gland will not heal.

Give an indication for Calcarea iodide.

Enlarged tonsils, where they are filled with little pockets, in scrofulous children who are weak, pale and fat.

In what special disease is Calcarea sulphurica indicated?

Suppuration of the tonsils.

Give the symptoms of Baryta carbonica in enlarged tonsils.

In scrofulous children, where every little cold starts up inflammation of the tonsils; the glands of the neck and behind the ear are swollen; it removes the predisposition to tonsillitis, and cures chronic enlargement of the tonsils.

When is Belladonna the Remedy?

The chief remedy for the swelling; the inflammation is deep, and there is a tendency to the formation of pus; the throat is bright red; sharp pains in tonsils.

When should Belladonna be changed for Hepar?

When pus forms and there are rigors, chills, sharp, sticking pains in tonsils, together with the throbbing.

How does Mercurius compare?

Pus has formed; the tonsil enlarges so as to hinder breathing; it favors the rapid formation and evacuation of pus.

Give indications for Bromine in tonsillar troubles.

Swollen tonsils, covered with network of dilated blood vessels; tonsillitis, with a feeling of rawness, accompanied by swelling of glands externally.

Mention three remedies, beside Baryta carb. and Calcarea iodide, that are useful for enlarged tonsils, and indications therefor.

Conium. No tendency to suppuration.
Lycopodium. Studded with small ulcers.
Hepar. Fish-bone sensation.

TUMORS.

Give uses for Calcarea fluorica in Tumors.

Knots, kernels or hardened lumps in the female breast, indurated glands of stony hardness, enlargements in the fasciæ and capsular ligaments of joints; felons.

What are the indications for Conium in Tumors?

Great hardness of the infiltrated glands, with flying stitches in them. Cancer, mammary tumors or beginning of scirrhus after contusions and bruises.

What remedy will sometimes cause the disappearance of fatty tumors?

Baryta carb.

What are some of the remedies for Epithelioma?

Conium, Hydrastis, Arsenic and *Clematis.*

What is an indication for Arsenicum in Cancer?

Sharp, lancinating pains.

TYPHOID FEVER.

Give the indications for Arsenicum in Typhoid Fever.

Late in the disease when the patient is faint, weak and exhausted, with cold sweat and delirium; the mouth and teeth are covered by sordes, the mouth is full of ulcers, there is diarrhœa, stools dark and offensive, intense fever and thirst.

What are some of the characteristic indications of Baptisia in this disease?

Typhoid conditions. The patient's mind wanders; he is restless and disturbed; he cannot sleep, and he thinks he is double or scattered about and he must move to get his pieces together again; there is great prostration; the back and limbs ache, and the patient feels bruised and tired all over; he is weak and faint.

How does the face look?

It has a heavy besotted look, as if drunken; the eyes are stupid and heavy.

What other symptoms would still further indicate Baptisia in Typhoid Fever?

High temperature and pulse, tenderness in the ileocœcal region, yellow, offensive stools; patient may be in a stupor and fall asleep while answering questions; brown, dark streak through the center of the tongue; all exhalations are offensive, sordes on the teeth, fetid breath, offensive urine and sweat.

How would Gelsemium compare with Baptisia in Typhoid Fever?

1. Both have muscular soreness and prostration.
2. Both have drowsiness and nervous excitement.
3. Both have feeling of expansion as if head and body were large.
4. Both have afternoon exacerbation of fever. The difference is simply one of intensity, *Gelsemium* being milder.

How does Rhus tox. compare?

The restlessness in *Rhus* is to relieve pain, and there is a triangular red tip to the tongue, and the discharges are not so offensive as under *Baptisia*.

Give in brief the indications for Bryonia in Typhoid Fever.

Soreness over the body; tired feeling; every exertion fatigues; he has a dread of all motion; a splitting, agonizing, frontal headache, worse from motion; the face gets red towards evening, nose-bleed in the morning, preceded by a fullness in the head; the sleep is troubled and the patient dreams of business, and there is high fever; delirium; patient wants to go home.

What are the indications for Arnica in Typhoid Fever?

Indifference to everything; they do not know or care that they are sick; go to sleep in answering questions; hot head, cool body and a bruised feeling all over the body; complains that the bed is too hard and tosses about to find a soft spot; involuntary stools and urine and petechiæ all over the body; ecchymoses and bed sores; later a condition of stupor in which the lower jaw drops.

What of the use of Gelsemium in Typhoid Fevers?

Sore, bruised sensations all over the body; early stages, dread of motion, drowsy, red face.

What are the indications for Muriatic acid in Typhoid Fever?

The tongue is dry and rattles in the mouth, there is a watery diarrhœa which is often involuntary while urinating, the patient is so weak that he slides down towards the foot of the bed; there is dropping of the lower jaw and cold extremities, the heart is feeble, irregular and intermits every third beat, bedsores, etc.

When would Nitric acid be indicated in Typhoid Fever?

When the stools are green, offensive and slimy, with hemorrhage from the bowels; fainting from least movement; threatened paralysis of the lungs, rattling breathing and intermittent pulse.

When should we give Opium in Typhoid Fever?

When there is profound congestion resulting from cerebral paralysis, loud stertorous breathing, dropping of the lower jaw, hot sweat—a bad omen—and high fever; sleepiness, with acute hearing, clocks striking and cocks crowing at a great distance keep patient awake.

What in brief are the symptoms that would indicate Rhus in Typhoid Fever?

Mild delirium, with desire to escape; great restlessness, with apparent relief from motion; answers questions slowly; frontal headache; dry, brown, cracked or red tongue, with triangular red tip; yellowish, brown, cadaverous and sometimes involuntary diarrhœa; pains in the limbs and a tympanitic abdomen.   Hydroa on upper lip.

Give the typhoid symptoms of Kali phosphoricum.

There is a dry tongue, brown in color, foul and putrid diarrhœa, great debility, low pulse, offensive breath, and sordes on the teeth; there is also great mental depression, delirium, etc.

Give symptoms indicating Carbo veg.

The vital forces seem exhausted; the patient is almost pulseless; feet and legs below knees are cold; there is present a dark brown, watery, horribly offensive stool.

Give symptoms calling for Lachesis.

Tongue trembles when protruded; catches on teeth; hemorrhages from any orifice of the body; dry and cracked lips; patient sensitive; dropping of lower jaw and involuntary discharges.

ULCERATION.

What is the character of the ulceration of Nitric acid?

The ulcers are irregular, deep and filled with exuberant granulations, bleed on slightest touch, have sticking pains in them and burn violently.

How does Mercurius differ from Kali bichromicum in ulceration?

The ulcers of *Mercurius* are rapidly spreading and superficial, while those of *Kali bichromicum* are circumscribed and deep with tendency to perforate.

What are some remedies having pimples, blisters or pustules surrounding ulcers?

Lachesis, Arsenic, Phosphorus, Lyc., Mercurius, Hepar, and *Silicea*.

What is characteristic of the Lachesis ulceration?

The great sensitiveness when touched, the blueness, and the bad odor.

Give indications for Arsenicum.

Burning, lancinating pains; ulcers bleed easily; the discharge is excoriating, dark and sanious.

What is the principal characteristic of the ulcers calling for Asafœtida?

Their extreme soreness being intolerant of all dressings.

What three remedies have ulcers about the small joints of the fingers?

Borax, Mezereum and *Sepia*

What is the ulceration of Carbo veg.?

Varicose ulcers of low type, flat ulcers discharging a thin ichorous pus, which is burning and offensive; the burning is worse at night.

URINARY DISORDERS.

What are the characteristic urinary symptoms of Apis?

Urine scanty or suppressed, with general œdema and drowsiness, lack of thirst and suffocation on lying down. Albuminous urine with tube casts.

What has Asparagus been used for?

Cystitis, enlarged prostate and catarrh of the neck of the bladder.

In what urinary trouble is Belladonna frequently indicated?

Involuntary urination during sleep in children.

Give the urinary symptoms of Benzoic acid.

Irritable bladder, with dribbling of strong-smelling urine; it is high colored and of a very offensive ammoniacal odor, like that of the horse.

What are the kidney symptoms of Berberis?

Sticking, tearing pains in the renal region; worse from deep pressure. The pains extend down the back, and down the ureters into the bladder; the back feels stiff and numb and the pains radiate from the kidneys to it.

Continue and give bladder symptoms of Berberis.

Cutting in the bladder, extending down the urethra; burning pain on urinating; the urine is yellow, turbid and flocculent, with whitish or red sediment; tearing pains in the bladder.

Give in brief the urinary symptoms of Cantharis.

Persistent and violent urging to urinate, with great tenesmus; the urine is passed only in drops, and seems like molten lead passing through the urethra; intense burning on urination, and aching in the small of the back.

Give the bladder symptoms of Causticum.

Paralysis of the bladder; involuntary urination while coughing; nocturnal enuresis of children during the first sleep.

Give two other drugs that have involuntary spurting of urine during coughing.

Squilla and *Natrum mur*.

What are the indications for Chimaphila in urinary disorders?

Catarrh of the bladder, with offensive, turbid urine and great difficulty in commencing to urinate.

What are the urinary symptoms of Digitalis?

Strangury and frequent urging to urinate; urging at night from enlarged prostate; relief from lying down; thick, yellow discharge from the urethra; useful in gonorrhœa.

What are the urinary symptoms of Equisetum?

Eneuresis, with marked vesical irritation, cystitis, painful urination and urging; bladder sore and tender; great desire to pass water from pressure on the bladder.

Give the indications for Eupatorium purpureum in the vesical irritation of women.

Dysuria, frequent painful urging with either excessive or scanty flow of urine, which is high colored and contains mucus; there is also aching in the region of the kidneys.

What are the symptoms of Ferrum phosphoricum in the urinary sphere?

Incontinence of urine from weakness of the sphincter, constant dribbling of urine during the daytime.

What is there characteristic about the urine of Ignatia?

It is very profuse and pale.

Give indications for Kali phosphoricum in Eneuresis or wetting the bed.

Where it is due to a paralytic or paretic condition of the bladder or from nervous debility; there is inability to retain the urine.

What are the urinary symptoms of Lycopodium?

The urine is turbid and bad smelling and deposits a red sand; child cries before passing water on account of lithic acid in the urine, the diaper is stained yellow.

What are the urinary symptoms of Nitric acid?

The urine smells as strong as a horse's urine; burning, tenesmus, and a sensation as if sticks were in the urethra when urinating.

What are the urinary symptoms of Nux?

Painful, ineffectual efforts to pass urine, with scanty discharge and burning; strangury, dribbling of urine in old people from enlarged prostate.

What are the characteristic symptoms of Pareira brava?

Constant urging to urinate, with pain in the glans penis and down thighs; patient sometimes has to get down on all fours to urinate, the straining is so severe; urine passes in drops and contains much thick and viscid mucus.

Give the chief use of Petroselinum.

A sudden desire to urinate, which if not attended to at once causes severe pain; children dance up and down and cry when this desire seizes them.

What effect has Phosphorus on the kidneys?

It produces a marked nephritis, with profuse discharge of bloody urine which contains casts.

What are the urinary symptoms of Sepia?

Irritable bladder, involuntary escape of urine during first sleep. Red sediment in the urine which is acid and fetid.

What effect has Stramonium upon the urinary secretion?

It causes suppression of the urine, and has been found of use in suppression of urine in typhoid fever.

What are the chief symptoms of Terebinth?

Dull, aching pains in the renal region; drawing pains and distressing strangury; urine scanty, bloody, dark and smoky looking and smelling like violets; there may be also excessive tympanites.

What symptoms call for Uva ursi?

Burning, scalding urination; urine stops suddenly, as if a stone had rolled in front of the internal orifice of the urethra. Urine is ropy and bloody.

Give indications for Opium.

Retention of urine from fright and after parturition.

What other drugs have retention of urine after labor?

Hyoscyamus, *Causticum* and *Arsenicum*.

What drugs produce suppression of urine?

Stramonium, *Zingiber*, *Lycopodium* and *Pulsatilla*.

What are the urinary symptoms of Hepar?

There is atony of the muscular coats of the bladder. The urine is voided very slowly by drops instead of a stream, and it takes a long time to empty the bladder. Nocturnal enuresis.

What are the indications for Pulsatilla in Cystitis?

Frequent urging to urinate, as if the bladder were too full; urine turbid. A useful remedy for cystic symptoms during pregnancy.

What is a peculiar symptom of Kreasote?

The patient urinates while dreaming of the act.

VERTIGO.

When is Conium indicated in Vertigo?

When due to cerebral anæmia; numb feeling in brain, as if stupefied; worse turning over in bed.

What is there characteristic about the Vertigo of Ferrum?

It comes on on going down hill, or on crossing water, even though the water is smooth.

Give Vertigo of Theridion.

Worse when closing eyes, and it is greatly aggravated by noise.

What other remedies have Vertigo worse when closing eyes?

Lachesis and *Moschus*.

What is the Vertigo of Causticum?

It is that occurring in the incipiency of paralysis; there is a tendency to fall forwards or sideways, and the sight is bedimmed.

When is Rhus tox. indicated?

In the vertigo of old people, which comes on when the patient rises from a sitting posture with heavy feeling in the limbs.

What is the Vertigo of Digitalis?

Of cardiac origin, the blood supply to brain being deficient. There is palpitation, breathlessness, feeble pulse, and a tendency to syncope.

VOMITING.

When is Æthusa cynapium indicated in Vomiting?

Vomiting in children of large and sometimes green curds of milk, *followed by great exhaustion;* there is a drawn look about the mouth suggestive of nausea. It may also be found useful in thin, yellow-green diarrhœa, preceded by cramps. Gastro-intestinal catarrh.

What is the vomiting of Antimonium crud.?

Vomiting from an overloaded stomach; from indigestible substances or rich, fat food; it comes on as soon as child eats or drinks; the vomited matters contain food or curdled milk.

When is Apomorphia useful in Vomiting?

When it is reflex from brain; vomiting of cerebral origin. In the vomiting of pregnancy it has achieved some success in the 30th trituration.

What other drugs have Vomiting of cerebral origin?

Bell., *Glonoine* and *Rhus*.

What drug has the symptom that as soon as water becomes warm in the stomach it is vomited?

Phosphorus.

What is the vomiting of Bismuth?

It comes on immediately after eating, with great pain.

What drug has vomiting of food three or four hours after eating?

Kreasote.

Mention a drug having vomiting of milk as soon as taken.

Calcarea carb.

When should Ipecac be given?

When there is intense nausea; vomiting comes on after eating. Nausea is even more characteristic than vomiting.

Give indications for Nux.

Nausea and vomiting after a debauch; everything eaten is vomited at once.

WHOOPING COUGH.

When is Drosera indicated in Whooping Cough?

Barking cough that comes so frequently that the patient cannot get his breath; worse in evening; efforts to raise the phlegm end in retching and vomiting.

What indications has Mephitis in this disease?

Whooping cough, with a marked laryngeal spasm and a whoop; cough is worse at night on lying down; there is a suffocative feeling, and the child cannot exhale.

How does Corallium rubrum compare?

Whooping cough, with smothering before the cough, and great exhaustion afterwards; the child gasps and gasps, and becomes black in the face. "Minute gun" cough, short, quick and ringing.

Give indications for Coccus cacti, another animal remedy, in Whooping Cough.

Paroxysms of cough, with vomiting of clear, ropy mucus, extending in great long strings even to the feet. Sensation as of a thread in the throat.

How does the expectoration differ from that of Kali bich.?

The *Kali bich.* expectoration is yellow, not clear albuminous.

Give the indications for Tartar emetic in Whooping Cough.

Cough worse when the child is angry, or when eating; it culminates in vomiting of mucus and food.

What is the Whooping Cough of Ipecac?

Convulsive cough, where the child stiffens and becomes pale or blue and loses its breath; great nausea and relief from vomiting.

What remedy is complementary in Whooping Cough and Convulsions?

Cuprum.

WOMEN, DISEASES OF.

What are the main characteristic female symptoms of Sepia?

The menses are usually late and scanty, though they may be almost any combination ; there are bearing down pains in abdomen ; must cross limbs to prevent protrusion ; there is extreme weakness, a dragging, weak feeling in the back ; the womb often feels as if clutched and suddenly released ; gone feeling in abdomen ; there are symptoms of uterine stasis.

When is the best time to give Sepia?

It comes in most usually after other drugs. Hering called it "a finishing remedy."

How does Lilium tigrinum resemble Sepia?

It has bearing down, everything seems to protrude, and is relieved by pressing the hand against the vulva. The ovarian and uterine pains are more intense than in *Sepia;* the nervousness is more marked and exercise relieves ; uterus is sore and sensitive ; patient is better when busy.

How does Lilium compare with Sepia as to time of aggravation?

Lilium is worse in the afternoon, *Sepia* in the forenoon.

What drug produces a soreness in the womb, a "consciousness of a womb?"

Helonias.

Give some other characteristic symptoms of Helonias.

Tired, aching feeling with burning in back and legs; there is also profound melancholy; soreness and weight in womb.

How does Sulphur resemble Sepia in its uterine symptoms?

There is the bearing down and the weak feeling or "goneness" in the abdomen and flushes of heat. They are complementary.

Give differentiation between Sepia and Murex.

The principal difference lies in the fact that *Murex* causes sexual excitement and copious secretions, otherwise the drugs are very similar. *Murex* has a feeling as if something was pressing on a sore spot in the pelvis. Secretions, such as menses and urination, are profuse.

What other drugs besides Murex produce sexual excitement?

Lilium tig. and *Platina*.

Differentiate between Sepia and Kreasote in female symptoms.

Both have intermittent menses.
Both have dragging down pains in back.
Both have pressure outward on genitals.
Both have painful coitus.
Both have red sediment in urine.
Both have turbid and offensive urine.

Kreasote has copious menses, *Sepia* scanty.

Kreasote has dragging in back relieved by motion, *Sepia* is worse from motion.

The *Kreasote* leucorrhœa is acrid and irritating, excoriating the parts, this *Sepia* does not have.

How does Stannum differ from Sepia?

It has prolapsus with bearing down and melancholy, but it has characteristically falling of the womb during hard stools. The patient is so weak that she cannot talk, and has to sit down several times while dressing in the morning.

How is Nux distinguished from Sepia?

Nux has a predominance of gastric symptoms; there is no "goneness" as in *Sepia;* there is less bearing down and dragging.

How does the action of Aloes on the uterus compare with Sepia?

The relaxation of tissues is more pronounced under *Aloes;* the heaviness, weight and dragging down are more intense; bowel symptoms will decide; there is loss of control of rectum and looseness of bowels.

How does Podophyllum compare here?

There is diarrhœa, and prolapsus and burning in pelvic regions; there is bearing down as if the genitals would protrude during stool. It differs from *Sepia* in its gastric symptoms.

What are the characteristics of Pulsatilla in uterine affections?

There is chilliness; there is heaviness and weight in pelvic regions. The menses are delayed and scanty; the flow is fitful and changeable; worse in warm room and better in open air; amenorrhœa after wet feet.

How is Pulsatilla distinguished from Sepia?

Pulsatilla is mild, tearful and whimsical.

Sepia is depressed, easily excited and irritable.
Pulsatilla—blondes.
Sepia—brunettes.

What are the female symptoms of Aurum?

Aurum congests the uterus and it becomes prolapsed from weight; there is a bruised pain in uterine region.

What are the main characteristics of Platina?

There is profuse and clotted menstrual flow occurring too early; voluptuous irritation of genitals and nymphomania; there is prolapsus and induration of uterus; ovaries are sensitive and have burning pains in them.

What drug cures nymphomania from worms crawling into vagina and there causing irritation?

Caladium.

Mention another drug which has dark, clotted menses, and how is it recognized?

Crocus; recognized by the symptom of a sensation as if something alive were moving about in the abdomen.

Give two drugs that have menses of bright red, partly clotted blood.

Sabina and *Millefolium.*

What other drug besides Sepia has induration of the cervix?

Carbo animalis; distinguished from *Sepia* by throbbing headache which follows menses.

What two drugs have the symptom that the womb seems as if pushed up when the patient sits?

Natrum hypochlorosum and *Ferrum iod.*

What are the characteristic female symptoms of Actea racemosa?

It is especially a remedy for threatened miscarriage when the pains shoot across the abdomen from side to side. Suppressed, tardy or irregular menstruation when accompanied by reflex disturbances.

How does Caulophyllum compare here?

It produces a spasm of the uterus and is useful in dysmenorrhœa; there is a sensation as if the uterus were congested, with fullness and tension in the hypogastric region. Menstruation too profuse and too frequent; the flow is passive.

What are the female symptoms of Senecio ?

The menses are scanty; there is apt to be associated with it bladder pains and dysuria; suppression of flow causes cough with bloody expectoration; sleeplessness reflex from uterine irritation.

Give female symptoms of Aletris.

With all uterine troubles and leucorrhœa there is extreme constipation, great effort being required for an evacuation; patient is weak and tired.

In what condition is Hydrastis indicated?

Prolapsus uteri with ulceration of the cervix; catarrh of uterus, with thick, yellow, tenacious discharge.

What drugs have a sensation in the groin as if sprained ?

Ammonium mur., Apis, and *Arnica.*

What are the female symptoms of Apis?

Amenorrhœa, congestion to head, with bearing down pains; great awkwardness.

What is the characteristic indication for Mel. cum sale.?

Feeling of soreness across the hypochondrium from ilium to ilium, in prolapsus uteri or chronic metritis.

What are the female symptoms of Cantharis?

Nymphomania, with the bladder symptoms; menses too black, too early, and too profuse; it favors the expulsion of moles, hyadids, etc.

What are the menstrual symptoms of Lachesis?

Menses scanty and feeble, black and offensive, with pain in the hips and bearing down in the left ovary; better when flow is established.

What drugs have especially sensitiveness to Coitus?

Platina, Sepia, Belladonna, Kreasote, Ferrum, Natr. mur., Apis and *Thuja*.

What are the uterine symptoms of Palladium?

Soreness in abdomen with downward pressure; tired feeling in back; knife-like cutting pains in uterus; swelling and pains in ovarian region; bearing down relieved by rubbing.

Give female symptoms of Alumina.

Chlorosis with pale and scanty menses and craving for indigestible substances.

What are the symptoms of the female system calling for Belladonna?

Bearing down, worse lying down, relieved by standing; menses bright red; painful congestive dysmenorrhœa; offensive menstrual flow, without apparent cause.

In this bearing down how does Sepia compare?

It has relief from lying down and is worse from standing, being the reverse of *Belladonna*.

What drug has bearing down worse from rest and relieved by motion?

Kreasote.

What symptoms has Bryonia on the female organs?

Vicarious or suppressed menstruation, flow dark and profuse; sharp sticking pains with the splitting headache of drug.

What are the menses of Calcarea carb.?

Early and profuse.

What are some female symptoms of Michella?

Engorged cervix with irritation at the neck of the bladder.

What are the symptoms calling for Gelsemium?

When the uterus feels as if squeezed by a hand; scanty flow; aphonia and sore throat during menses.

Give female symptoms of Graphites.

The womb feels as if it would press out of the vagina; enlargement of left ovary with scanty delayed menses; anteflexions and anteversions; dysmennorrhœa of fat women with herpetic eructions, patients constantly cold.

What are the characteristic symptoms of Natrum mur. in female affections?

There are scanty menses, painful coitus and red sediment in urine. Menses may be scanty for a day or two then copious; the sadness of the drug is increased before the menses. When the patient gets up in the morning she must sit down to prevent prolapsus. Backache and morning aggravation are characteristics.

What is the menstruation of Conium?

Late and scanty.

What are some other female symptoms of Conium?

Mammæ lax and shrunken or become enlarged and painful. Fibroid tumors of the uterus, induration of cervix, ovaritis with lancinating pains; itching around pudenda—ill effects of suppressed sexual instinct.

What are the indications for Secale in uterine hemorrhage?

Persistent hemorrhages of dark, thin blood. It is a passive flow and it may be offensive. There may be coldness, formication and tingling.

How does this compare with Bovista?

Bovista has bright, thin hemorrhage; it is very periodic. The flow chiefly occurs at night or in the morning.

Give the hemorrhage of Ustillago.

The flow is bright red, partly clotted. Slight manipulations, such as examinations, cause hemorrhage. Menorrhagia from retroflexions.

What drug has dark, thick uterine hemorrhage, and menstruation occurring chiefly at night?

Magnesia carb.

What drug has menses flowing only in daytime when about on feet?

Causticum.

What are the hemorrhages of Trillium?

Bright red, profuse hemorrhages, with faintness in abdomen. It is an active acute hemorrhage, with pains in sacroiliac synchondroses.

How does Millefolium compare here?

It is a remedy for thin, bright red flow.

What is the metrorrhagia of Sabina?

Bright red, paroxysmal, with pains in limbs. Uterine hemorrhage at change of life.

Ipecac has the same symptoms as Sabina, how is it distinguished?

By the nausea.

What drug has early and scanty menses in tall, slender females?

Phosphorus.

What are the female symptoms of Kali carbonicum?

Menses are too early and too profuse, and last too long; there may be itching of the body during menstruation and a great deal of backache. Amenorrhœa, with backache.

What are the female symptoms of Calcarea fluor?

In excessive menstruation with bearing down pains, flooding; displacements of the uterus; prolapsus; dragging pains in the region of the uterus and in the thighs.

Give three remedies having early and profuse menstruation, stating how they may be distinguished.

Belladonna. Menses too early and too profuse, with downward pressure as if everything would protrude, bright red in color, or of decomposed, dark red blood, which feels hot to parts.

Calcarea carb. Too early, profuse, and last too long in characteristic Calcarea patients; the feet feel cold and damp.

Nux vomica. Too early and profuse; nausea in the morning during menses, with chilliness and pressure towards the genitals.

Distinguish three remedies having early and scanty menstruation.

Conium is one of the principal remedies for early and scanty menses, accompanied by painful cramps in abdomen, preceded by soreness or nodular swellings of the breast.

Silicea. Menses early and scanty; the discharge has an acrid smell; cold feet during menses; burning soreness and itching of the pudenda.

Phosphorus. Early and scanty menses, preceded by leucorrhœa.

WORMS.

What are the symptoms calling for Cina in worm affections?

Sickly, pale face, with rings around the eyes; gritting of the teeth at night; canine hunger, or variable appetite; the child picks its nose and cries out in its sleep; jerking of hands and feet; urine milky.

In what intestinal condition is Natrum phosphoricum indicated?

In intestinal worms, either long or thread worms, with symptoms of acidity, picking at the nose, squinting and twitching of the facial muscles.

What indications has Spigelia in worm affections?

Strabismus, jerkings with paleness of the face, blue rings around the eyes, faint, nauseated feeling and colic about the navel.

How does Stannum act as a vermicide?

According to Hahnemann it so stupefies the worms that purgatives would dislodge them at once.

What is a useful remedy for pin worms?

Teucrium; there is much itching about anus, capricious appetite, picking of nose, offensive breath, disturbed sleep and general restlessness.

YELLOW FEVER.

In what disease is Crotalus most often indicated?

In yellow fever, in the stage of black vomit, where there is low delirium, yellow skin, and oozing of blood from every orifice of the body.

What remedy is said to be a preventive of Yellow Fever?

Carbo veg.

When is Argentum nitricum the remedy?

When there are signs indicating hemorrhage from gastric mucus membrane; patient sinks and vomiting becomes worse.

Give indications for Arsenicum.

Vomiting of brown, turbid matter mixed with mucus or blood; great prostration and restlessness.

When is Lachesis indicated?

Brown tongue, tender abdomen, dark vomit, urine almost black; trembling tongue with brown coating on teeth.

INDEX.

Abortion—See Miscarriage	179
Abscess	1
Ars.	3
Bell.	1
Calc. carb.	3
Calc. iod.	3
Calc. sulph.	1, 2
Calcium sulphide.	1, 2
Carbo veg.	3
Hepar sulph.	1
Lach.	2
Merc.	2
Rhus.	3
Silicea	2
Sulph.	3
Acne	3
Ant. tart.	4
Ant. crud.	4
Aurum	4
Hepar sulph.	4
Kali brom.	4
Ledum	4
Natr. mur.	4
Phos. ac.	4
Sanguin.	4
Sulph.	3
After Pains	4
Arn.	5
Bell.	5
Caul.	5
Cham.	5
Cimicif.	5
Croc.	5
Gels.	5
Puls.	5
Xanthox.	5
Agalactia	5
Agnus cast.	5
Bell.	5
Calc. c.	5
Cham.	5
Puls.	5
Ricinus com.	5
Urtica urens	5
Alcoholism	6
Ars.	6
Hyosc.	6
Lach.	6
Nux	6, 7
Opium	6
Ranunc. b.	7
Stram.	6
Sulph.	7
Sulph. ac.	7
Amenorrhœa	7
Acon.	7
Apis	8
Bell.	7
Bry.	8
Calc. c.	7
Cimicif.	8
Dulc.	8
Ferr.	8
Graph.	9

INDEX.

Lyc. 7
Natr. mur. 9
Opium 7
Phos. 8
Puls. 8
Sep. 9
Sulph. 9
Verat. 7

Anæmia 9
Alumina 10
Calc. phos. 9
Cinchona. 9
Ferr. acet. 10
Ferr. met. 9
Ferr. phos. 10
Graph. 10
Natr. mur. 10
Puls. 9

Angina Pectoris 10
Amyl nitr. 11
Ars. 11
Cimicif. 10
Gelsem. 11
Glon. 11
Kalmia. 11
Nux. vom. 11
Tabacum 11
Spigelia. 11

Aphonia—See Hoarseness . 136

Aphthæ—See Mouth, Diseases of. 180

Apoplexy 12
Arn. 12
Bell. 12
Gelsem. 12
Hyosc. 12
Lach. 12
Opium 12

Appendicitis 12
Bell. 12

Bry. 13
Ferr. phos. 13
Kali mur. 13
Lach. 13
Rhus. 13

Asthma. 13
Ammoniac gum 13
Apis 14
Arsenicum 13
Brom. 15
Carbo veg. 15
Grindelia 15
Ipecac 14
Kali bich. 14
Lobelia 14
Natr. sulph. 14
Nux vom. 15
Pothos. 15
Stram. 14
Zingib. 15

Backache 15
Æsculus 15
Anac. 17
Calcar. fluor. 15
Cannabis Ind. 17
Cobalt 17
Conium. 17
Kali carb. 17
Kali phos. 16
Ledum 17
Nux v. 17
Oxalic ac. 16
Petrol. 17
Phos. 16
Rhus. 16
Ruta. 17
Secale 17
Sepia 17
Staph. 17
Sulph. 16

Zinc	17	Zinc	22

- Boils 18
  - Arn. 18
  - Bell. 18
  - Calc. carb. 18
  - Calc. sulph. 18
  - Hepar. 18
  - Lach. 18
  - Lyc. 18
  - Sil. 18
  - Sulph. 18
- Bones, Diseases of 19
  - Asa 19
  - Angustura 20
  - Aur. 20
  - Calc. fluor. 19
  - Calc. phos. 19
  - Fluor. ac. 19
  - Phos. 19
  - Platina mur. 20
  - Silicea 19
  - Stillingia 20
  - Strontiana c. 20
  - Symphytum 20
- Brain, Diseases of 20
  - Acon. 20
  - Bell. 20
  - Carbo an. 21
  - Cinchona 21
  - Glon. 20
  - Hyosc. 21
  - Kali brom. 21
  - Nux vom. 21
  - Phos. 21
  - Phos ac. 21
  - Picric ac. 21
  - Rhus. 21
  - Spigel. 21
  - Stram. 21
  - Sulph. ac. 21
  - Verat. vir. 22

- Bright's Disease—See Kidneys, Diseases of .. 147
- Bronchitis 22
  - Acon. 22
  - Ammon. carb. ... 22
  - Ant. tart. 24
  - Baryta c. 24
  - Balsam Peru. 23
  - Bell. 22
  - Bry. 23
  - Carbo veg. 23
  - Caust. 23
  - Chel. 24
  - Ipec. 23
  - Kali bich. 24
  - Kali carb. 24
  - Kali sulph. 25
  - Lyc. 24, 25
  - Natr. mur. 22
  - Pix. liq. 23
  - Phos. 25
  - Sang. 25
  - Sulph. 25

- Cancer—See Tumors. ... 238
- Carbuncle 26
  - Anthracin 26
  - Ars. 26
  - Carbo veg. 27
  - Lach. 26
  - Rhus 26
  - Tarentula 26
- Chlorosis—See Anæmia .. 9
- Cholera Asiatica 27
  - Acon. 28
  - Ars. 28
  - Camph. 28, 29
  - Carbo v. 27
  - Cupr. 27, 29
  - Hydrocy. ac. 28

Jatropha	28
Secale	28
Veratr.	28
Cholera Infantum	**29**
Acon.	29
Aethusa.	31
Arg. n.	29
Ars.	29
Bell.	29
Bismuth	29
Calc. c.	30
Calc. phos.	30
Cham.	31
China	31
Crot. tig.	30
Elater.	30
Ferr. phos.	30
Ipec.	30
Mercurius	32
Podo.	30
Psor.	31
Sulph.	31
Veratr.	31
Chorea	**32**
Agar.	32
Caust.	33
Cimicif.	32
Ignatia	32
Magnes. phos.	32
Mygale	32
Stram.	32
Tarentula	32
Zincum	33
Zizia	32
Climacteric Disorders	**33**
Amyl nitr.	33
Cimicifuga	33
Glon.	33
Lach.	33
Sang.	33

Colds and Catarrhal Affections	**34**
Acon.	34
Allium c.	35, 37
Ammon. c.	39
Ammon. mur.	39
Ars.	34, 35, 36, 37
Ars. iod.	40
Arum.	35, 37
Aur.	39
Brom.	39
Bry.	42
Camph.	34
Cham.	37
Cycl.	37
Cinnabar.	40
Dulc.	42
Elaps.	41
Euphras.	35, 37
Ferr. phos.	36
Gels.	34
Hydras.	37, 38
Hep.	39
Kali bi.	37, 38
Kali c.	38
Kali hyd.	36, 37
Lach.	40, 42
Lyc.	35
Merc.	34, 36, 37
Nitr. ac.	39
Natr. c.	41
Natr. m.	36, 37
Nux v.	36
Penthorum	37, 38
Phos.	35, 41
Puls.	37
Rhus	45
Sabad.	32
Sang.	41
Sambucus	40
Sinapis	37

INDEX.

Spigel 38
Sticta 40
Teucrium 41
Verbascum 40
Wyethia 41

Colic 42
   Alumina 43
   Alum. 43
   Bell. 43
   Cham. 44
   Coloc 42, 43, 44
   Cupr. 43
   Diosc 42
   Ipec. 44
   Magnes. phos. 43
   Natr. sulph. 43
   Nux vom 43
   Opium. 43
   Platina. 43
   Plumbum 43
   Staph 44
   Verat 44

Constipation 44
   Alumina 45
   Ammon. mur. 47
   Anac. 45
   Bry. 39–44
   Caust 48
   Carbo v. 46
   Graph. 46
   Hydras. 48
   Lyc. 45–46
   Magnes. mur. 48
   Natr. mur. 47
   Nux vom. . . . 44, 45, 46
   Opium 44
   Phos. 47
   Platina 47
   Plumb. 45–48
   Selen. 48

Sepia 47
Sil. 47
Sulph. 41
Veratr. 44, 48

Convulsions 49
   Bell. 49
   Cham. 49
   Cina 49
   Cocc. 49
   Cupr. 49
   Glon. 49
   Hydrocy. ac. 50
   Hyoscy. 50
   Ign. 50
   Ipec. 50
   Secale 49
   Stram. 50
   Verat. 50

Coryza—See Colds and Catarrhs 34

Coughs 51
   Acon. 53
   Ambr. g. 56
   Antim. t. 51
   Aralia 51
   Brom. 51
   Bry. 51
   Bell. 51–54
   Calc. c. 53
   Caust. 52–55
   Cupr. 55
   Con. 54, 55
   Cocc. cact. 53
   Corall. r. 53
   Dros. 52
   Eup. p. 52, 56
   Hep. 54
   Hydrocy. ac. 56
   Hyosc. 54–55
   Ignat. 53

Kali bi. 55
Kali sulph. 56
Lach. 54
Laur. 55
Lyc. 52
Magnes. phos. 55
Meph 53
Nitr. ac. 56
Natr. mur. 52
Opium 54
Phos. 51–52
Rumex. 52, 54
Sepia 56
Spong. 56
Sil. 52
Squilla 52, 55
Sticta 54
Verbasc. 57
Croup 57
Acon 57
Ant. t. 58
Brom. 51–57
Chlor. 52–58
Hepar 51–58
Iodine 57
Kali bi. 52–58
Kaolin 52–58
Sambucus 52–58
Spong 57
Cystitis—See Urinary Disorders 243

Debility 59
Ars. 59
Cinchona 59
Cocculus 59
Colch. 60
Mur. ac. 59
Phos. 59
Phos. ac. 59
Sulph. ac. 59

Delirium 60
Absinth. 60
Bell. 60
Hyosc. 60
Phos. 60
Stram. 60
Verat. 60
Delirium Tremens—See Alcoholism 6
Dentition 61
Bell 61
Ferr. phos. 61
Calc. phos. 61
Cham. 61
Kreas. 61
Diabetes 62
Ars. 62
Lactic ac. 62
Phos. ac. 62
Uran. nitr. 62
Diarrhœa 62
Acon. 62
Ars. 64
Apis 63
Arg. n. 63
Aloes 63–66
Arn. 64
Apoc. c. 63
Bell. 65
Borax 65
Bry 66
Calc. ac. 67
Calc. carb. 65
Calc. phos. 65–71
Carbo v. 64–70
Cham. 65
Chel. 71
Chin. 64, 67
Coloc. 69
Colch. 72

INDEX. 269

Crot. tig.	68
Diosc.	69
Dulc.	72
Elat.	68
Euphorb.	72
Ferr. phos.	71
Ferr. met.	64–67
Gamboge	63
Gels.	64, 70
Geranium	69
Gnaphalium	69
Gratiola	68
Hepar	65
Hyosc.	71
Ipec.	70
Iris	69
Jatropha	69
Kali brom.	69
Kali bi.	66
Lach.	70
Lept.	70
Lith. carb.	70
Magnes. carb.	65, 66
Merc.	65, 71
Natr. mur.	72
Natr. phos.	71
Natr. sulph.	66
Nitr. ac.	70
Nux vom.	70
Nuphar	69
Œnothera	69
Oleander	67
Opium	64
Opuntia	69
Petrol	69
Podo.	66, 67–68, 71
Phos.	63
Paulinia	69
Psor.	71
Phos. ac.	67, 72
Puls.	64–69
Rhus	70
Rheum	65
Rumex	66
Secale	64
Staph.	65
Silicea	71
Sulph.	66, 71
Thuja	72
Veratr.	64–68
Diphtheria	73
Alcohol	74
Ailanthus	74
Arum triph.	74
Apis	73
Ars.	73
Bapt.	74
Brom.	75
Kali bi.	73
Kali perman.	73
Lac. can.	73
Lach.	74
Lyc.	75
Merc. bin.	74
Merc. cyan.	74
Merc. prot.	74
Mur. ac.	75
Nitr. ac.	75
Phytolacca	75
Dropsical Affections	75
Acet. ac.	76
Apis	76
Apoc. can.	76
Ars.	76–77
Dig.	76
Lach.	77
Lyc.	77
Dysentery	77
Acon.	77–78
Aloes	77
Ars.	77
Canth.	78

Caps.	77
Carbo v.	78
Cinchona	78
Ferrum phos.	78
Merc. sol.	78
Merc. corr.	78
Nux vom.	78
Dysmenorrhœa	78
Bell	78
Borax	80
Cactus	79
Caul.	79–80
Cham.	79
Cimicif.	79
Magnes. phos.	79
Puls.	79
Viburnum	79
Xanthox.	80
Dyspepsia—See Gastric Derangements	95
Ear, Diseases of	80
Aur.	82
Bell.	80
Borax	81
Caps.	82
Carbo an.	82
Caust.	80
Cham.	81
Dulc.	81
Ferr. phos.	80
Graph.	82
Hepar.	82
Kali mur.	81
Lach.	81
Nitr. ac.	82
Phos.	81
Psor.	81
Puls.	81
Sil.	82
Eczema—See Skin Diseases of	213
Eneuresis—See Urinary Disorders	243
Epilepsy	83
Argentum nitr.	84
Artemesia	83
Bufo rana.	84
Calc. carb.	84
Cicuta	82
Cina.	84
Cupr.	83
Hydrocy. ac.	83
Hyosc.	83
Indigo	84
Nux vom.	83
Œnanth croc.	83
Sil.	83
Epistaxis–See Hemorrhages	116
Erysipelas	85
Apis	85
Bell.	85
Canth.	85
Euphorb.	85
Lach.	85
Rhus	86
Stram.	86
Eye, Diseases of	86
Acon.	91
Allium cepa	89
Ammon. gum.	91
Apis	86
Arg. n.	86
Ars.	90, 92
Asaf.	92
Aur.	86
Bell.	86, 88, 91
Bry.	92
Calc. carb.	92
Canth.	87

Caust. 87, 90	Sulph. 94
Cinnabaris 87	Veratr. vir. 93
Comocladia 87	Fissure of Anus 94
Euphrasia 87	Graph. 94
Ferr. phos. 87	Nitr. ac. 94
Gelsem. 87, 88, 90	Pæonia 94
Graph. 88	Ratanhia 95
Hepar 88, 90	Silicea 95
Kali bi. 88	
Kali hyd. 92	Gangrene 95
Kali mur. 89	Ars. 95
Kali sulph. 89	Carbo v. 95
Kalmia 90	Secale 95
Lach. 92	Gastric Derangement . . . 95
Lyc. 90	Abies can. 107
Merc. 89	Abies nig. . . . 96, 98, 108
Merc. corr. 89	Alumina 108
Natr. mur. 89	Anacard. 99, 101
Paris quad. 90	Angustura 104
Physostigma 88	Ant. cr. 100, 104
Phos. 90	Arn. 108
Puls. 90, 91	Ars. 99, 100, 106
Rhus. 86, 90	Arg. n. . . 100, 102, 104, 105
Ruta 91	Asa. 110
Spigel. 91	Bell. 109
Staph. 90	Bism. 103, 106
Silicea 90	Bry. 107
Sulph. 91	Cadmium 107
Thuja 91	Calc. carb. 107
Zinc 91	Calc. phos. 109
	Carbo v. 96, 97, 98, 99, 100, 104
Fever (Simple) 92	Carbo an. 102
Acon. 92, 93	Carbol. ac. 110
Apis 93, 94	Chelidon. 101
Ars. 93	China 98, 99, 104
Bell. 93	Colch. 102, 109
Bry. 94	Cycl. 109
China 94	Ferr. m. 108
Gels. 93, 94	Graph. 101, 104
Phos. 93, 94	Hep. 107
Puls. 93, 94	

INDEX.

Hydras. 105
Ign. 108
Ipec. 100, 105, 106
Iod. 104
Iris. 108
Kali bi. 96, 109
Kali c. 103
Kali mur. 109
Kreas. 96
Lach. 100
Lyc. 96, 97, 98, 99, 100, 104
Natr. carb. 96, 103
Natr. mur. 109
Natr. phos. 110
Natr. sulph. 103
Nux mosch. 96, 97
Nux vom., 95, 96, 98, 99, 101, 103, 104.
Petrol. 101
Phos. 102, 103
Puls. . . . 98, 99, 100, 105
Robinia 106
Salycil. ac. 110
Sep. . 96, 99, 102, 103, 105
Staph. 105, 106
Sulph. 96, 99, 102
Sulph. ac. 97, 106
Tabac. 104
Thuj. 100
Glandular Troubles . . . 110
Alumina 111
Badiaga. 111
Bell. 111
Brom. 111
Calc. c. 111
Carbo an. 111
Con. 111
Iod. 110
Spongia 111
Silicea 111
Gleet 111

Puls. 112
Sep. 112
Sulph. 111
Gonorrhœa 112
Arg. nitr. 112
Cannabis sat. 112
Canth. 112
Copaiva 113
Cubeba 112
Dig. 113
Gels. 113
Merc. 113
Merc. corr. 113
Natr. sulph. 113
Petroselinum 114
Puls. 114
Sulph. 114
Thuja 113
Gout 114
Ammon. phos. 114
Antimon. crud. . . . 115
Arn. 114
Benz. ac. 115
Bry. 115
Calc. carb. 115
Colch. 114
Guaiac. 115
Led. 115
Lith. carb. 115
Lyc. 115

Hay Fever 115
Ars. 115
Ranunc. bulb. . . . 115
Sabadilla 116
Sinapis nig. 115
Hemorrhages 116
Acalypha Ind. . . . 116
Acon. 118, 119
Ars. 119
Bell. 117

Bov.	117
Cact. gr.	119
Carbo veg.	116, 118, 119
Cinchona	116, 118
Cinnamom	118
Crocus sat.	119
Erigeron	118
Ferrum met.	118
Hamam.	119
Ipec.	117, 118
Lach.	117
Merc.	118
Millefol.	117, 118, 119
Phos.	116, 119
Sabina	117
Secale	116
Trillium	118
Ustillago	117

Hemorrhoids 119
    Æsculus 120
    Aloes 119
    Collinsonia 120
    Hamam. 120
    Nux 120
    Ratanhia 120
    Sulph. 120

Headache 121
    Acon. 125
    Ant. cr. 129
    Anac. 130
    Apis 129
    Arg. nitr. 123
    Aloes. 129
    Bell. . . 121, 123, 127
    Bry. 122, 126
    Cannab. Ind. 128
    Carbol. ac. 125
    Carbo an. 124
    Carbo veg. 122, 126
    Caust. 125
    Cocc. 122
    Coffea. 125, 129
    Cinchona. 123
    Cimicifuga 127
    Ferr. met. 129
    Gels. . . . 122, 125, 126
    Glon. 127
    Hep. 128
    Ignat. 125, 128
    Iod. 125
    Ipec. 126
    Iris v. 121, 125
    Juglans 122
    Kali bi. 128
    Lach. 128
    Melilotus. 123
    Menyan. 123
    Merc. 125
    Natr. carb. 128
    Natr. mur. 124, 125
    Natr. sulph. 129
    Nux vom. 122, 124
    Oleander 129
    Onosmod. 129
    Pallad. 127
    Paris 124
    Petrol. 122
    Phelland. 127
    Phos. ac. 130
    Psor. 125
    Puls. 130
    Rhus. 128
    Sang. 121
    Selen. 128
    Sep. 124
    Sil. . . . 122, 123, 125, 126
    Spigel. 122, 126
    Sulph. 125
    Therid. 124
    Thuja. 125, 126
    Verat. alb. 125
Heart, Affections of 130

Acon.	130
Adonis	135
Amyl nit.	135
Ammon. carb.	136
Actea rac.	131
Apis	136
Arn.	132
Ars.	132
Aur.	133
Cact.	133
Con.	133
Convall.	135
Dig.	131
Euphras.	133
Gels.	131
Grindel.	133
Graph.	134, 136
Glon.	135
Iod.	134
Kali bi.	134
Kali carb.	134
Kali hyd.	134
Kali nitr.	136
Kalmia.	130
Lach.	134
Lactuca.	134
Lycopus	135
Naja	135
Natr. mur.	136
Petrol.	136
Phos.	133
Phytol.	131
Puls.	130, 133
Rhus.	130, 131
Spigel.	132
Spong.	132
Sulph.	134
Tabac.	134
Veratr. vir.	133
Zinc.	133
Herpes—See Skin, Diseases of.	213
Hoarseness	136
Ammon. caust.	138
Argentum met.	138
Arum triph.	138
Carbo veg.	136
Caust.	136, 137
Eupator. perf.	137
Gels.	137
Graph.	136, 138
Phos.	137
Selen.	136
Senega.	137
Sulph.	136
Hydrocephalus	138
Apis	139
Apocyn.	139
Digitalis	139
Hellebore.	138
Sulph.	139
Hysteria	139
Apis	141
Asafoet.	139, 141
Castoreum	139
Ignat.	140, 141
Moschus	140
Nux mosch.	140
Platina.	141
Tarentula	140
Valeriana	140
Zincum valer	141
Influenza	141
Ars. iod.	142
Drosera	141
Dulcamara	142
Eupator. perf.	141
Gelsem.	142
Sabadilla	142
Injuries.	142

INDEX.

Arn. 142
Calendula 143
Con. 143
Hyper. 142
Ledum 143
Rhus 142
Ruta 143
Staph. 143
Sulph. ac. 143
Symphytum . . . 143
Insomnia—See Sleep, Affections of 221
Insanity—See Mental Conditions, etc. 165
Intermittent Fever . . . 144
Apis 144
Ars. 144
Caps. 144
Carbo veg. 147
Cinchona 144
Chinin. sulph. . . . 144
Cornus flor. 145
Eupator. perf. . . . 145
Ferrum met. 145
Gels. 145
Ignat. 145
Ipec. 145
Lach. 147
Natr. mur. 146
Natr. sulph. 146
Nux 146
Rhus 146
Iritis—See Eye, Diseases of . 86

Kidneys, Diseases of . . 147
Apis 148
Ars. 147
Berb. vulg. 148
Canth. 148
Digital. 148
Merc. corr. 147

Phos. 148
Terebinth. 148

Labor 148
Bell. 149
Caul. 149
Cham. 148
Cimicif. 149
Gels. 149
Puls. 150
Secale 149
Laryngitis 150
Acon. 151
Apis 151
Argent. met. 150
Ars. 151
Arum triph. 150
Bell. 151
Brom. 151
Chlorine 151
Gelsem. 151
Hep. 150
Lach. 151
Sambucus 151
Spong. 150
Leucorrhœa 151
Aletris 151
Bell. 152
Alumina 151
Borax 152
Calc. carb. 152
Calc. phos. 152
Graph. 151
Helonias 152
Hydras. 151
Kreas. 152
Lil. tig. 152
Puls. 152
Sepia 152
Stannum 152
Liver, Diseases of 153

INDEX.

Aurum 158
Berb. v. 156
Bry. 154, 155, 156
Carbo veg. 158
Carduus 157
Cham. 156
Chel. 155
Chionanthus 156
China 158
Dig. 155
Kali bi. 156, 157
Laur. 156
Lept. 153
Lyc. 154
Magnes. mur. 157
Merc. 153–154
Myrica 155
Natr. sulph. 157
Nux vom. 154
Podo. 154
Phos. 156, 157
Rhus. 154
Stram. 154
Sulph. 158
Tarax. 156
Yucca 154, 156
Locomotor Ataxia . . . 158
Alumina 158
Ammon. mur. 159
Argent. nit. 160
Cham. 159
Coloc. 159
Ferrum. 159
Kali brom. 160
Kali carb. 159
Lyc. 159
Phos. 159
Plumb. 159
Secale 159
Zinc. 159
Lumbago—See Backache . 15

Mammary Gland, Affections 160
of 161
Bell. 161
Bry. 161
Calcarea fluor. 161
Con. 160
Crot. tig. 160
Phellandrium 161
Phos. 161
Phytol. 160
Puls. 161
Silicea 161
Marasmus 161
Calc. carb. 162
Calc. phos. 161
Hepar 162
Iodine 162
Magnes. carb. 162
Natr. mur. 162
Measles 162
Acon. 163
Bry. 162
Cupr. 163
Gels. 163
Kali bi 163
Puls. 163
Stram. 163
Zinc. 163
Meningitis 164
Acon. 164
Apis 164
Artemisia 165
Baryta carb. 165
Bell. 164
Bry. 164
Calcarea carb. 165
Cupr. 164
Hell. 164
Zinc. 195
Menstruation—See Women,
Diseases of 251

Mental Affections	165
Acon.	165
Actea rac	178
Aur.	169
Alumina	172
Ambra	179
Anac.	167, 177
Ant. cr.	173
Apis	172
Arg. n.	174
Ars.	172
Bapt.	174
Bell.	165, 172
Bry.	168
Cann. Ind.	172
Calc. carb.	171
Caust.	175
Coffea	165, 175
Coloc.	169, 179
Cina	178
Cinchona	172
Cimicif.	178
Cham.	168
Con.	179
Croc.	175
Cypriped.	176
Dulc	166
Dig.	178
Gels.	173, 174
Glon.	176
Graph.	174
Hepar	169, 171
Hyosc.	166
Iod.	172, 176
Ign.	169, 170
Kali brom.	176
Kali carb.	176
Kali phos.	178
Lach.	166, 167, 171
Lil. tig.	177
Lyc.	171
Merc.	177
Natr. carb.	178
Natr. mur.	173
Nitr. ac.	168
Nux mosch.	177
Nux vom.	168
Opium	173
Paris	167
Pallad.	173
Petrol.	175
Phos.	175, 177
Phos. ac.	170, 173
Plat.	170
Puls.	169, 173, 177, 179
Rhus	173, 177
Sep.	169
Sil.	173
Staph.	168
Stann.	177
Stram.	166, 167
Sulph.	166, 171
Thuja	174, 175
Verat. alb.	166, 173
Valer.	169
Miscarriage	179
Acon.	180
Cham.	180
Cimicif.	179
Hamam.	180
Sabina	179
Secale	180
Viburnum	179
Mouth, Diseases of	180
Ars	181
Bapt.	180
Borax	180
Bry.	180
Lach.	181
Lyc.	181
Natrum hyp.	181
Merc.	180

INDEX.

Mur. ac. 181
Nitr. ac. 181
Phytol 181
Salicylic ac. 181
Mumps 181
   Bell. 181
   Merc. 182
   Puls. 181
   Rhus 181

Neuralgia 182
   Acon. 182
   Actea rac. 184
   Allium cepa 182
   Ammon. mur. 182
   Ars. 182, 183
   Bell. 182
   Caps. 183
   Cedron 182
   Cham. 183
   Cinchona 183
   Colch. 183
   Kalmia 184
   Kreas. 184
   Magnes. phos. 184
   Mezer. 183
   Platina 183
   Spigel. 183
   Stann. 184
   Thuja 184
   Verbasc. 183
Neurasthenia 185
   Phos. 185
   Phos. ac. 184
   Picric ac. 184
   Silicea 185
   Zinc. 185

Œdema of the Glottis—See
   Laryngitis. 150
Ophthalmia—See Eye, Diseases of 86

Orchitis 185
   Aur. 186
   Clem. 185
   Ham. 186
   Iod. 186
   Puls. 186
   Rhod. 185
   Spongia 186
Otitis—See Ear, Diseases of. 80

Ovarian Diseases 187
   Apis 187
   Arg. met. 187
   Ars. 187
   Colocynth 188
   Graph. 187
   Lach 187
   Pallad. 188
   Platina 187
Ozæna—See Colds and Catarrhs 34

Paralysis 188
   Acon. 188
   Caust. 188
   Dulc. 188
   Gels. 188
   Hepar 189
   Kalmia 189
   Plumb. 189
   Rhus 189
   Sep. 189
   Zinc. 189
Parotitis—See Mumps . . . 181
Peritonitis 189
   Ars. 190
   Bell. 189
   Bry. 189
Phthisis 190
   Ars. 192
   Ars. iod. 190
   Balsam Peru. 192

Calc. carb. 190, 191
Calc phos. 190
Carbo an. 191
Carbo veg. 191
Codeine 192
Laur 192
Nitr. ac. 190
Phos. 192
Sang. 192
Sil. 192
Spongia. 191
Stann. 192
Sulph. 191, 193
Tuberculin 191
Pleurisy 193
   Acon 193
   Apis 193
   Bry. 193
   Kali carb. 193
   Ranunc. bulb. 193
   Rumex 193
   Senega. 193
   Sulph. 193
Pleurodynia 193
   Actea rac. 194
   Acon. 194
   Bry. 194
   Gaultheria 194
   Ranunc. bulb 193
   Rhus rad. 194
   Rumex 194
   Senega 194
Pneumonia 194
   Acon. . . . 194, 195, 196
   Ant. t. 198, 199
   Bry. 196, 197
   Chel. 198
   Dig. 199
   Ferr. met. 197
   Ferr. phos. 195, 196
   Hepar 199

   Iod. 195
   Ipec. 199
   Kali carb. 197
   Kali mur. 196
   Lach. 199
   Lyc. 198
   Merc. 198
   Phos. 196, 197
   Sang. 195
   Sulph. 197, 197
   Veratr. vir. 195, 196
Pregnancy, Disorders of . . 199
   Acon. 200
   Actea rac. 200
   Bry. 200
   Caul. 201
   Cerium ox. 200
   Hamam. 201
   Lyc. 201
   Magnes. carb. 201
   Nux vom. 201
   Puls. 199, 200
Puerperal State, Affections
   of 201
   Acon. 201
   Actea rac. 201
   Bell. 202
   Cicuta 202
   Gels. 202
   Glon. 202
   Hyos. 202
   Kali brom. 202
   Opium 202
   Veratr. vir. . . . . . . 202.

Rheumatism 202
   Ammon. phos. 203
   Apis 207
   Arn. 208
   Actea rac. . . . 204, 208
   Actea spic. 204

INDEX.

Bell. 208
Benz. ac. 203, 206
Bry. 203, 204, 205
Caust. 205, 208
Calc. carb. 203, 208
Caul. 204
Cham. 206
Colch. 204, 205
Dulc. 206
Ferr. met. . . 203, 206, 207
Ferr. phos. 203
Guaiac. 204
Kalmia 205
Kali bi. 205
Kali hyd. 205. 207
Kali sulph. 205
Led. 203
Lyc. 203
Lith. carb. 203
Magnes. carb. 207
Nux mosch. 207
Puls. 203, 205
Ranunculus bulb. . . . 205
Rhus . . . 202, 204, 206
Rhod. 203
Ruta 208
Sang. 207
Sil. 207, 208
Sulph. . . . 205, 206, 208
Sulph. ac. 208
Verat. 206
Viola od. 205

Scarlet Fever 208
Ail. 208, 209
Apis 210
Bell. 209
Bry. 209
Lach. 210
Muriatic acid 210
Rhus 209

Zinc. 209
Sciatica 210
Ammon. mur. 211
Coloc. 210
Gnaphalium 210
Kali bi. 210
Kali hyd. 210
Phytol. 211
Rhus tox. 211
Scrofula 211
Calc. carb. 212
Graph. 212
Iod. 211
Merc. 212
Silicea 212
Sulph. 211
Seasickness 212
Apomorphia 213
Cocculus 213
Petroleum 212
Skin, Diseases of 213
Ammon. carb. 218
Anac. or. 216, 218
Anac. oc. 218
Ant. cr. 218
Ant. tart. 220
Apis 213, 217
Arc. lappa 216
Arn. 219
Ars. 215, 218
Ars. iod. 218
Bell. 217
Caust. 218
Calc. carb. 217, 219
Canth. 213
Chin. sulph. 214
Comoclad. 219
Crot. tig. 213, 218
Dolichos 219
Dulc. 219
Graph. 215, 217

INDEX.

Grindelia 218
Hepar 220
Hippomane 220
Hydrocotyle 220
Hura 214
Kali brom. 218
Kreas. 217
Lyc. 215
Mez. 214, 215, 216
Natr. carb. 221
Natr. mur. 217
Nux juglans 216
Oleander 216
Petroleum . . . 216, 217
Pix liq. 221
Psor. 214
Ranunc. b. 214
Ranunc. sc. 214
Rhus 213, 218
Sarsap. 220
Sep. 217
Sil. 220
Staph. 216
Sulph. 215
Tellur. 217
Terebinth. 217
Thuja 218
Urtica ur. 217, 220
Vinca 216
Viola tric. 216, 220
Sleeplessness 221
Ambra 221
Bell. 221
Cham. 221
Cocc. 222
Coffea 221
Cypripedium 221
Ferr. phos. 222
Gelsem. 223
Ignatia 221
Hyoscy. 222
Nux 222
Puls. 222
Sulph. 222
Sore Throat. 223
Ammon. caust. 223
Arg. nit. 227
Alumina 226
Bapt. 223
Bell. 223
Canth. 223
Caps. 223
Carbo veg. 227
Cistus can. 223
Ferr. phos. 224
Gels. 224
Guaiac. 224
Hepar. 229
Ignat. 224
Kali bi. 224
Kali mur. 224
Lach. 225
Lyc. 225
Merc. 225
Merc. bin. 225
Merc. corr. 226
Merc. prot. 225
Natr. mur. 226
Nux 226
Nitr. ac. 226, 227
Phytol. 226
Sulph. ac. 226
Spermatorrhœa 227
Agnus cast. 227
Bufo. 227
Calad 227
Calc. carb. 229
Con. 227
Eryngium. 227
Gels. 228
Lyc. 229
Nuphar 228

Nux vom.	228	Stillingia	233
Phos.	228		
Phos. ac.	228	Teeth, Affections of	234
Picric ac.	228	Cham.	234
Selen.	229	Coff.	234
Staph.	229	Hepar.	234
Sulph.	229	Kreas.	234
Zinc.	229	Lach.	234
		Merc.	234
Spinal Irritation	229	Silicea	234
Actea rac.	230	Staph.	234
Agar.	229		
Chinin. sulph.	230	Tetanus	235
Cocc.	230	Acon.	236
Natr. mur.	230	Angustura	235
Phos.	230	Bell.	236
Physostigma	230	Cicuta	236
Zinc	230	Curare.	235
		Hydrocy. ac.	236
Spleen, Diseases of	231	Hypericum	236
Aranea diad	231	Passiflora	235
Ceanothus	231	Physostigma	235
Cinchona	231	Phytolacca	235
Chinin. sulph.	231	Pictrotoxine	235
Grindelia	231	Silicea	336
		Stram.	235
Sunstroke	231	Strychnia	235
Glon.	231	Veratr. vir.	236
Lach.	232	Throat—See Sore Throat	223
Natr. carb.	231	Tonsillitis	236
Synovitis	232	Baryta carb.	237
Apis	232	Bell.	237
Bry.	232	Brom.	237
Sulph.	232	Calc. iod.	236
		Calc. sulph.	237
Syphilis	232	Con.	237
Carbo an.	233	Hepar.	237
Hepar	233	Lyc.	237
Kali hyd.	233	Merc.	236, 237
Lach.	233	Sil.	236
Lyc.	233		
Merc.	232, 233	Tumors.	238
Merc. protiod.	232	Ars.	238
Nitr. ac.	233		

INDEX.

Baryta carb. 238
Calc. fluor. 238
Clematis 238
Con. 238
Hydras. 238

Typhoid Fever 238
   Arn. 240
   Ars. 238
   Bapt. 239
   Bry. 240
   Carbo veg. 241
   Gels. 239, 240
   Kali phos. 241
   Lach 241
   Mur. ac. 240
   Nitr. ac. 240
   Opium 241
   Rhus 329, 241

Ulcers and Ulceration . . . 242
   Ars. 243
   Asa. 242
   Borax 242
   Carbo veg. 243
   Hepar. 242
   Lach. 242
   Lyc. 242
   Merc. 242
   Mez. 242
   Nitr. ac. 242
   Phos. 243
   Sep. 242
   Sil. 242

Urinary Disorders 243
   Apis 243
   Asparagus 243
   Ars. 247
   Bell. 243
   Benz. ac. 243
   Berberis 243
   Canth. 244

   Caust. 244, 247
   Chimaphila. 244
   Digital 244
   Equisetum 244
   Eupator. purp. 244
   Ferr. phos. 245
   Hepar. 247
   Hyos. 237
   Ignat. 245
   Kali phos. 245
   Kreas. 247
   Lyc. 245, 247
   Natr. mur. 244
   Nitr. ac. 245
   Nux vom. 245
   Opium 246
   Pareira. 245
   Petros. 246
   Phos. 246
   Puls. 247
   Sep. 246
   Squilla 244
   Stram. 246, 247
   Terebinth 246
   Uva ursi 246
   Zingiber 247

Vertigo 247
   Caust. 248
   Con. 247
   Dig. 248
   Ferr 247
   Lach. 248
   Mosch. 248
   Rhus. 248
   Therid. 247

Vomiting 248
   Æthusa. 248
   Antim. crud. 248
   Apomorphia. 449
   Bell. 249

Bismuth.	249
Calcarea carb.	249
Glonoine	249
Ipecac.	249
Kreasot.	249
Nux	249
Phos.	249
Rhus	249

Whooping Cough 249
    Coccus Cacti 250
    Corall. rub. 250
    Cuprum 250
    Drosera 249
    Ipecac 250
    Kali bich. 250
    Mephitis 250
    Tartar emet. 250

Women, Diseases of, . . . 251
    Actea rac. 255
    Aletris 255
    Aloes 253
    Alumina 256
    Ammon. mur. 255
    Apis 255, 256
    Arnica 255
    Aurum 254
    Belladonna . 256, 257, 260
    Bovista 258
    Bryonia 257
    Caladium 254
    Calc. carb. 257, 260
    Calc. fluor. 260
    Cantharis 256
    Carbo. an. 254
    Caulophyllum 255
    Caust. 259
    Cimicifuga 255
    Conium 258, 260
    Crocus 254
    Ferrum met. 256
    Ferrum iod. 256
    Gelsem. 257
    Graphites 257
    Helonias 251, 252
    Hydrastis. 255
    Ipecac. 259
    Kali carb. . . . 259
    Kreas. 252, 256, 257
    Lach. 256
    Lilium tig. 251, 252
    Magnesia carb. 259
    Mel. cum. sale. 256
    Michella 257
    Millefol. 254, 259
    Murex 252
    Natr. hyp. 254
    Natr. mur. 256, 258
    Nux vom. 253, 260
    Palladium 256
    Platina . . . 252, 254, 256
    Phos. 259, 260
    Podo. 253
    Puls. 253, 254
    Sabina 254, 259
    Secale 258
    Senecio 255
    Sepia . 251, 252, 253, 254, 256, 257
    Silicea 260
    Stannum 253
    Sulphur 252
    Thuja 256

Worms 261
    Cina 261
    Natr. phos. 261
    Spigel. 261
    Stann. 261
    Teucrium. 261

Yellow Fever 262	Carbo veg. 262
Arg. nitr. 262	Crotalus 262
Arsen. 262	Lach. 262

ESSENTIALS

OF

Homœopathic Therapeutics;

BEING A

QUIZ COMPEND

OF THE

APPLICATION OF HOMŒOPATHIC REMEDIES
TO DISEASED STATES.

A COMPANION TO THE

Essentials of Homœopathic Materia Medica.

ARRANGED AND COMPILED ESPECIALLY FOR THE
USE OF STUDENTS OF MEDICINE.

BY

W. A. DEWEY, M. D.,

Professor of Materia Medica in the University of Michigan, Homœopathic Medical College. Former Professor of Materia Medica, Hahnemann Hospital College, of San Francisco, Cal. Associate Author of *The Twelve Tissue Remedies of Schussler*, Author of the *Essentials of Homœopathic Materia Medica*. Member of American Institute of Homœopathy, California State Homœopathic Medical Society, Homœopathic Medical Society of the State of New York, Homœopathic Materia Medica Society of New York, etc., etc.

SECOND EDITION, REVISED AND ENLARGED.

B. Jain Publishers (P) Ltd.

USA — EUROPE — INDIA

**ESSENTIALS OF HOMEOPATHIC THERAPEUTICS
BEING A QUIZ COMPEND**

7th Impression: 2020

All rights reserved (including all translations into foreign languages). No part of this publication may be reproduced, stored in a retrieval system, or transmitted in any form or by any means, electronic, mechanical, photocopying, recording or otherwise, without the prior written permission of the publisher.

© Copyright with the Publisher

Published by Kuldeep Jain for
B. JAIN PUBLISHERS (P) LTD.
D-157, Sector-63, NOIDA-201307, U.P. (INDIA)
Tel.: +91-120-4933333 • *Email:* info@bjain.com
Website: **www.bjain.com**
Registered office: 1921/10, Chuna Mandi, Pahargani,
New Delhi-110 055 (India)

Printed in India by
J.J. Offset Printers

ISBN: -978-81-319-0121-2